To our amazing subscribers, the
inspiration for this Guide.

-Kelsey and Kendra Murrell

TABLE OF CONTENTS

THE
GLAMTWINZ GUIDE
TO LONGER, HEALTHIER HAIR

KELSEY AND KENDRA MURRELL

FOREWORD

I will never forget the day I laid eyes on Kendra and Kelsey. I don't remember the year, but I do remember the medium - YouTube. Two perfectly coiled brown beauties with long, lush curls and flawless makeup demoing how to Style Your Hair. Simply STUNNING! I knew I had to work with them. They have since recorded a host of YouTube videos for CURLS, reviewed almost all of our products and have even made CURLS appearances. I can say, I have never seen anything like the line to meet the GlamTwinz! Each and every naturalista, hoping to replicate their style, wanted to take a piece of them home.

Luscious locks and the GlamTwinz go hand and hand, so penning the "GlamTwinz Guide to Longer, Healthier Hair" was a natural progression. They have effortlessly created a well-documented, systematic approach for caring for, and growing beautifully healthy, natural hair. From the easy to grasp steps and real confessionals, to the "don't get it twisted" myth buster section and the "girlfriend to girlfriend tone" – the "GlamTwinz Guide to Longer, Healthier Hair" is a clear winner! I plan to see it on the bestsellers list soon.

Naturalistas, now you can take the GlamTwinz home with you!

Mahisha Dellinger
CURLS Beauty Brand
Founder & CEO

INTRODUCTION

Yes, anyone can grow LONGER, HEALTHIER HAIR!

The good news is, ALL hair grows. Of course, hair grows at different rates and in different growth cycles, but all hair grows. One person might easily grow her hair to neck length and another might just as easily grow her hair to bra-strap-length, but all hair grows. For instance, our hair used to grow to armpit length easily. After that point, maintaining length was harder. We learned the key to retaining length was properly caring for our texture of hair.

Now, to the bad news—some people may just have to work harder than others to achieve their hair goals. If you're not retaining length, you are simply not caring for your roots –OR– you are neglecting your ends (chances you are dealing with breakage at the ends of the hair). Technically, the bad news isn't bad at all. Working harder to retain more length for your strands will empower you to understand and care for the uniqueness of your hair.

Don't be discouraged. With a good hair care regimen, anyone can retain length. Once we understood what made our hair unique – started treating our ends like friends, eliminating relaxers, and implementing "no-heat-summers" – we began to see tremendous growth.

After six years of hair growth, we can tell you the work gets a bit easier and the process is well worth it!

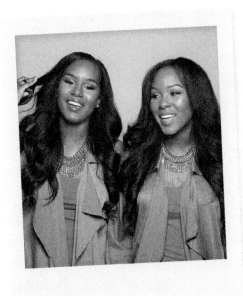

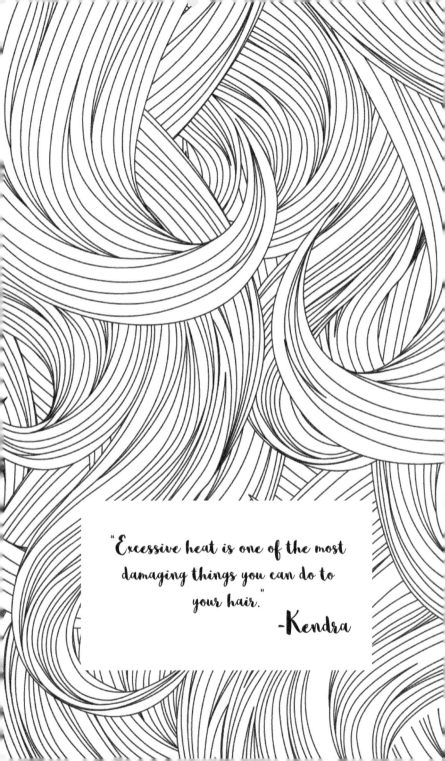

"Excessive heat is one of the most damaging things you can do to your hair."

-Kendra

CHAPTER 1:
NO HEAT

We know what you're thinking! You were so excited about reading our Guide to Longer, Healthier Hair—that is until you turned the page to Chapter One and read the words, No Heat! Yes, we said it, "No Heat!" So, don't forcibly pinch yourself, this is not a dream . . . don't vigorously blink your eyes, you are not hallucinating . . . don't continually rub your lids, you are seeing straight . . . and [for heaven's sake] don't close the book . . . YOU CAN DO THIS.

If you enjoy styling your hair often, the words No Heat! can be downright scary. We are well aware that a world without flat irons, curling wands, and blow dryers seems intolerably petrifying. We get it. Using heat to style hair provides versatility, eliminates frizz, and creates sleekness. Unfortunately, that sleek shine is only temporary because using constant heat (especially at high levels) is likely the worst part of any daily or weekly hair routine. The good news is, while using excessive heat is probably the most damaging thing any girl can do to her hair, eliminating heat is perhaps the easiest step she can take toward treating her damaged hair and ultimately achieving maximum length.

Think About It

If you use 400° or more of heat on your hair, seven days a week, your hair endures nearly 3,000° of heat weekly. That's nearly ten times the amount of heat you would use to bake a cake, roast a hen, or broil a chicken. You are literally cooking your hair. Why not heat an oil-filled frying pan on the stove and swirl your hair around in the grease?

Continuous heat will only make your hair straw-like and brittle. High temperatures can strip your hair of much needed moisture, alter its natural curl pattern, modify its thickness, and destroy your delicate ends. As you'll learn in Chapter One, preserving healthy ends is a major component of growing and maintaining long healthy hair. Each of these reasons is why excessive heat is potentially the MOST damaging action in hair care and the reason why No Heat! is the first tip in our book. If heat usage is a major barrier for you, you are not alone. We know about the effects of cookin' hair all too well.

Kendra's Confession

During my last year of middle school, Kelsey and I began going to the salon less and treating our own hair more. We convinced our mom that if she would spend just a little extra on hair products and styling instruments now, we would save her a ton of money later. We sealed the deal with a promise that we would grow our shoulder-length hair to waist length if she provided the right resources. After months of convincing, she finally agreed. It was a promise that we can now say we kept, but there were some bumps in the road along the way.

One of the first styling tools she purchased for us was a top-of-the-line flat iron. It was the best straightening tool out at the time, and we had to have it. The very first time I used it, I fell in love. My hair had never looked better. In addition to being bone-straight, it had body, shine, and volume. The iron and I instantaneously became best friends. I visited him and experienced his magical powers every single day, sometimes multiple times a day. Regrettably, the start of my daily visits with my newfound friend quickly became the end of my luscious, healthy locks.

During that time, everyone was wearing straight hair, and I was no exception. I went through a short period (literally, just a few weeks) when I constantly used heat on my hair. After getting my monthly treatment at the salon, which included a heat-enhanced deep conditioning treatment, a dryer-induced roller set, and a style-completing flat iron, I began applying additional heat to my strands. Throughout the day, every day, I touched up my edges.. . my ends . . . and my strays. I was fanatic about achieving the perfect look, and as far as I was concerned, it was necessary to apply heat daily in order for my hair to look good.

I was a heat addict. My mom and sister continuously warned me about my excessive use of heat. Though they tried to warn me, my only response to their intervention was, "I know what I'm doing." After all, no one used a flat iron better than me. I was the Lebron James of straightness and style, and my hair looked phenomenal for the first couple of weeks. It was only after about a month or so that I realized my Rookie-of-the-Year status would be short-lived.

I began to see the physical difference in the condition of my hair. My hair became unbelievably dry. The dryer it got, the more strays would appear. So, naturally, I would apply additional heat to tame the fly-aways. The more heat I applied, the more brittle the hair became, so I would condition, blow-dry, and flat iron again. It was a never-ending cycle.

Eventually, I was unable to bandage the damage, and my mom demanded I revisit the salon.

I will never forget my cosmetologist's words: "Your hair is unrepairable, I have to cut the damage off." Cut the damage off? What did she mean, cut it off? Couldn't a hot oil treatment and some deep conditioning fix the problem? I was devastated. I listened carefully as she explained that heat-damaged hair was treatable, but not repairable.

As it turns out, I had suffered a LOT of breakage, and the amount of hair on the floor after my reparative cut was evidence of the severity of my actions. As I watched my newly cut strands fall to the floor, I knew the oath I had made to my mom had fallen with it. I could not believe this was happening to me. I literally cried, and after returning home with collar-bone length hair my mom quietly collected every single flat iron and curling rod in the house and while I can't say for sure, each is likely at the bottom of the city dump.

This was a huge wake-up call for me and it helped both my sister and I reevaluate how often we should use heat on our hair. I hope my story and Chapter 1 of this book are a huge wake-up call for you. If you are a heat addict, STOP NOW!

If you're thinking, "I'm natural, so my hair can stand the heat," or, "My hair looks good to me and I use a flat iron three times per week," trust us, even if you don't notice the damage right away, you're going to see it over time. Both of those theories are two of the biggest myths about heat and hair. First, simply because chemicals are not used regularly in your hair, doesn't mean your unprocessed hair is better suited for high levels of constant heat. Chemical usage should not be substituted with heat usage. It doesn't matter whether you apply color, perms, or relaxers, an excessive heat user will end up having long-term damage if you continues to apply daily heat.

Second, if your hair is incredibly strong and appears healthy despite excessive usage of high levels of heat, chances are you are not seeing incredible hair growth. Your hair may look healthy, but achieving growth beyond your "natural length" will be nearly impossible. Let's consider one strand of hair. As the hair cuticle sprouts beyond the scalp, it's a baby strand. This strand is new to the world of pollutants, styles, and heat. Soon after it sprouts, you begin flat ironing twice a week at high levels of heat. Since it's the first time the strand has been exposed to heat, it's not a big deal, particularly if you have been blessed with incredibly thick hair. As the hair grows, the next week, you repeat the process. The portion of the hair that has just penetrated the scalp is now experiencing heat for the first time, but your newly formed end is experiencing repeated heat for the third and fourth time. Two weeks later, the hair grows a fourth of an inch, and you repeat the same process. Now, the newest portion of the strand is experiencing heat for the first time, the portion that grew in two weeks ago feels the heat effect for the second time, and the oldest piece receives a triple whammy. Eventually, the strand grows out to shoulder length.

At this point, you have applied heat countless times, and you apply it just once more. Although you may not see hair fall off the strand while using the flat iron, at this point the strand is incredibly brittle and weak. During the day, you run your fingers through your hair or comb your strands. Inconspicuously, the end of the strand simply breaks off. Since the hair is not breaking off in clumps, you don't notice it. Yet, loss of that end and the hundred thousand other ends of hair on your head is likely the reason you are not able to see actual growth—because your "natural length" is also your "breaking point". Even if you don't notice the damage right away, in time you'll see it.

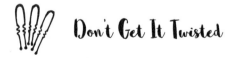 Don't Get It Twisted

We are in no way advocating TOTAL elimination of heat on your hair. Truthfully, total heat elimination is likely not the best for your hair because some heat is beneficial. For instance, hot oil treatments can create remarkable results for dry or damaged hair, and a proper deep conditioning treatment requires low levels of heat to maximize results.

In fact, when we are not in a no-heat-phase, we use heat (blow drying and flat ironing) two to four days out of each month. This means we flat iron twice a month and sometimes curl once during the weeks in between. Our heat usage is on a schedule, and our hair has been trained to withstand that usage. For example, when we are wearing straight hair, we wash, blow-dry, and flat iron on days one and fourteen. During these weeks, we implement heatless deep conditioning. Then, the flat irons are retired until the next scheduled use. Between flat irons, we allow ourselves one curling-induced style. We might wand, curl, or roll. Then, the curling tool is put away until the next scheduled use. Additionally, each time we apply heat to our hair, we use medium heat. (Thicker hair may require more heat, and finer hair may require less heat. When using heat, apply the appropriate amount of heat for your texture of hair to maximize desired results.)

The following illustration demonstrates our heat usage over a thirty-day cycle.

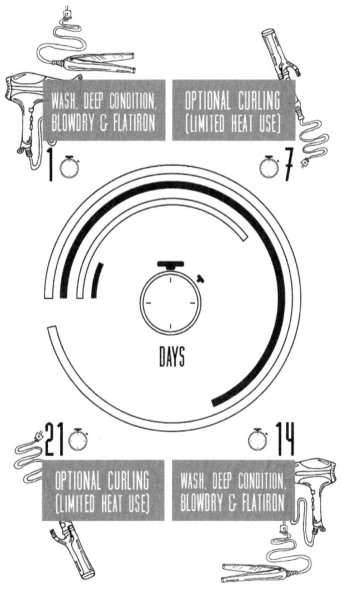

WASH, DEEP CONDITION, BLOWDRY & FLATIRON

1

OPTIONAL CURLING (LIMITED HEAT USE)

7

DAYS

21

OPTIONAL CURLING (LIMITED HEAT USE)

14

WASH, DEEP CONDITION, BLOWDRY & FLATIRON

21

What we are promoting is minimizing overuse of heat. Anything over 450° of direct heat is damaging, and repeated use of such levels of heat is detrimental. The bad thing about heat is that the damage it causes is long-term. Revitalizing the hair after experiencing heat damage can be an arduous task. Our hair and heat routine was developed through trial and error. Chances are yours will too, because hair type and cuticle texture predetermines the amount and temperature of heat that is good or hazardous to your hair.

Challenge Yourself

Minimizing heat usage is not as hard as you may think. Let's see how much discipline you have. Consider NO HEAT soon. Give yourself a set time and slowly reduce your heat usage. For instance, if you're used to using heat once a week, start by using it once every two weeks. If you are using heat once every two weeks, try once a month. You get the picture. Slowly decreasing heat usage over time will create easily attainable goals. The less heat, the better.

In addition to decreasing overall heat usage, we implement no-heat-summer. Simply put, we commit ourselves to wearing our natural curls approximately four months out of the year. Those warmer summer months give our hair the time it needs to thicken, grow, and repair itself. The process gives us major results! Plus, our natural curls are perfect for the heat, sweat, and humidity that accompany the summer months. Maintaining straight hair in the summer is not an easy task, so why not go without it for a while?

At the start of fall, we straighten our locks and gauge the change in length. After the first straightening we were floored at the amount of growth we achieved during the prior summer. Every summer since has produced similar results. This plan works incredibly well for us. We consistently achieve extreme growth during our curly months, sometimes 3 or more inches.

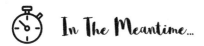 In The Meantime...

Don't worry, you don't have to be a master cosmetologist to learn about other things that you can do to your hair in lieu of heat and straightening. We understand that many people have a hard time styling their hair without the use of heat—especially if heat has been your primary styling tool. This dilemma is completely understandable. Here is our suggestion. The best way to avoid too much heat is to start a routine. Routines train the hair to do what you want it to do on a weekly basis.

Hair reacts well to a routine. So, pick a day to do your hair, whether it's once a week or every two weeks. Whatever your routine may be (washing, conditioning, blow drying, etc.), make the day you choose the only day you use heat. Then, maintain that style for a period of time, and commit the remaining time period as "unheatable."

The best way to learn heatless styling techniques is simple – just do it! If you become disciplined enough to master Tip #1, the rest of the instructions in this book will come incredibly easy. If you will remain patient and demonstrate consistency, minimizing heat usage will maximize your potential for growth. Not only will you unlock unprecedented levels of length, you might unlock a mountain of treasure exploring the world of protective styling.

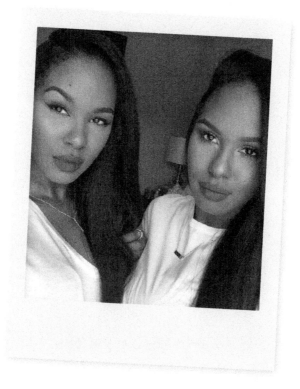

"If you want to wear your hair down, that's where twist outs and braid outs come in."

-Kelsey

CHAPTER 2:
PROTECTIVE STYLING

Dying of hair boredom . . . can't put down the hot tools . . . or are you simply one of those people who likes to try new things with your hair? If you answered, "yes," to any of these questions, then this is the chapter for you. Of course, we do NOT want to sound like one of those hour-long infomercials filled with empty promises in exchange for your hard-earned dollar, but it's true . . . protective styles are the perfect alternative to heat styling. No gimmicks! Protective styles provide exactly what they promise—a style that acts as a defense for your hair.

Think About It

Let's say you're a hair-down-kind-of-girl. Whether it's curly or straight, you always wear your hair down. In fact, it's highly likely that your friends don't remember the last time they saw your hair in a ponytail, bun, or braid. On a typical day, the alarm buzzes at 6 a.m. You yawn, roll over, and silence the alarm. In the bathroom, if your hair is curly, you moisten, moisturize, and finger comb; and if your hair is straight, you brush, part, curl, or straighten. You check your perfectly flowing hair in the mirror and think, "Yeah, you look good girl!" You leave the bathroom, and dress yourself, pulling your favorite shirt over your head. The cotton fibers strip a bit of moisture from your hair, and a few strands get caught in the stylish buttons that trim the shoulder of the shirt. While you step into your pants, lace your shoes, and scarf down your breakfast, you run your fingers through your hair six, maybe seven times (hey, we know . . . it's a habit that's hard to break).

Before you leave you throw your jacket over your head, around the top half of your body. Unfortunately, before the jacket properly rests on your shoulders a couple of strands get caught in the zipper. Afterward you grab a scarf and throw it around your neck and the section of your hair that covers your neck is now engulfed beneath the scarf and out the door you go.

When you open the front door, a gust of wind blows your way. It's cold! Instinctively, you run your hands through your hair to secure your perfected style. While in transit, you rest your head on the seat of the train or Uber. When you arrive at your destination, a girlfriend compliments your hair, running her fingers through your strands. While you're grateful for the compliment, she just repositioned your style, so you run your fingers through the hair again to reinforce its position.

While working, you twist the ends of your hair repetitively (yeah, another bad habit). After lunch, you visit the ladies room and finger comb/brush your hair. Then, when you leave work, it begins raining . . . We could literally go on, and on, and on. By the day's end, your hair has been brushed, combed, curled, straightened, pulled, buttoned, zipped, covered, blown, scrubbed, rubbed, curled, twirled, and rained on. Need we say more? Loose hair demands constant manipulation. It's no wonder you have a hard time maintaining those ends. They aren't just frizzy, they are trying to run away for dear life!

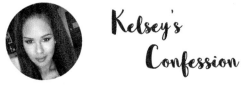

Kelsey's Confession

I accidentally discovered the benefits of protective styling. I was in high school. I was trying to transition my hair, and my mom was trying to teach us responsibility. So, she politely suggested (like over and over again) that we get a job, start saving, and contribute to our monthly car insurance premium, increasing fuel expenses and constant weekend outings. Of course, Kendra and I were in school and our schedules were exhausting.

We were up early to prep for school, endured a long school day, completed evening work hours, and fulfilled our homework obligations. I loved my newly-forming curly hair, but I had very little time to maintain it. While Kendra would spend additional time maintaining her hair, I spent that extra time tucked comfortably under my sheets. As a result of my unfamiliar, tiresome schedule, I would wear the same bun for a week or more. Buns were so easy. Simply put, they were a big time saver. I would wash, condition, and bun my hair on Sunday. Then, Monday through Saturday, I would wrap a silk scarf around it at night and unwrap it in the morning.

Once, when I was *extra* tired, I actually wore the same bun for two whole weeks! Initially I thought I'd regret my lack of hair maintenance. Nonetheless, the day I took my hair down, the texture was wonderfully different and I noticed it had maintained a lot of moisture. When I let my hair fall, I immediately, noticed it looked longer, shinier, and healthier. More surprisingly, after washing and measuring my strands, I discovered my hair had grown TWO INCHES in just two short weeks! *Two inches in two weeks? I was on to something!*

For the remainder of the year, I decided to continue this routine for two weeks out of every month—and it paid off. I always saw the most hair growth when I was bunning. Needless to say, buns became a big contribution to my hair growing process. I was giving my hair a break for weeks at a time. Ultimately, my strands thanked me for the hiatus. If you've ever been to our YouTube channel, you know I enthusiastically endorse protective styles and the benefits they provide.

It is surprising to know how many of our subscribers think that the best way to achieve the prettiest, presentable and most stylish looks require heat or loose hair. The notion is another widely received fallacy in the world of hair. If you sincerely believe that your beauty is enhanced solely through heat-based styling, big curls, or loose strands, you clearly haven't discovered the world of protective styles.

Creative protective styles are classy, versatile, fun, and sexy! The possibilities are endless.

When it comes to protective styles, here are three basic styles:

Buns

As Kelsey's confession reveals, buns are a girl's best friend. Once you learn to perfect your favorite bun, you diversify it by making it high, low, or lopped. You can also manipulate buns by making them messy and fun or tidy and chic. You can also try top knots, which are a show stopper. No matter which combination of technique you use, buns are simple, they save time, (and most importantly) they provide protection.

Twist Outs & Braid Outs

Next, twist outs and braid outs are another awesome way to protect the hair from heat, weather and manipulation. Additionally, if you just can't resist wearing your hair down, it's a good way to wear your hair down without applying heat. Twist and braids create relaxed patterns in the hair, locking in moisture and improving health. Even better, with twist outs and braid outs, you can look hot while reducing heat. Plus, they are the perfect way to help train, form, or change your natural curl pattern. So, if you happen to not have naturally textured hair or curly hair, these styles provide great alternatives for you to mix-it-up!

Braids

Lastly, the braid. Braids have been around since forever. We'll bet your great granny used them and her great, great grandma before that. That's because, when done properly, braids can be an incredible benefit to your hair. They imbed applied moisture, create wonderful textured patterns, protect the length of the hair, and secure the ends of the hair. Also, there are so many variations of braids to try.

Rope braids, dual textured braids, halo braids, waterfall braids, spiral braids, and chain link braids are among the many braids to try. The notorious French braid is classic and simple, and if you're feeling ambitious or creative go for a fishtail braid. Before bedtime, the traditional pigtail braids can be used to achieve those sexy beach tail waves the following day. These are small tips that can increase the benefits of braids. For instance, prior to doing your bedtime braids, you should apply leave-in conditioner spray if necessary to reactivate the hair shaft in order to achieve those desired waves.

CAUTION: Although braids are entrenched with benefits, improper installation can create detriments. Braids must be done properly. When hair is braided too tightly, it can cause thinning, alopecia, and receding hairlines.

Those are the basics. When it comes to daytime and nighttime protective styles, buns and braids are a girl's BFF. Both styles can be manipulated into cute and chic looks on any face. Moreover, braid outs and twist outs can break the monotony of hair training. Plus, all of these styles are lifesavers on those dirty hair days and each will help you achieve your "long, healthy hair goal" while still looking stylish and cute. If you master the basics of these three styles, you can achieve hundreds of variations of protective styles. All of these styles will help you achieve your goals of long, healthy hair while still looking chic and stylish. For more information or tutorials on any of these styles, just check out our YouTube channel.

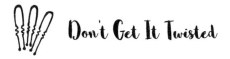 # Don't Get It Twisted

We are not saying that protective styling is the only way to grow long healthy hair. As we mentioned in Chapter 1, some people have longer hair cycles and can grow long hair easier and quicker. Kendra prefers lower maintenance styles. Nevertheless, through a well-fashioned hair routine, she's trained her hair to require low manipulation. That has worked well for her.

What we are saying is that protective styling can provide great benefits. Particularly, protective styles can help you if:

· You do not grow long hair easily
· You have short hair growth cycles
· You constantly grow your hair to a certain length and fail to see more growth beyond that point
· You simply want to grow your hair longer than you ever have.

If you are one of the women in the preceding categories, protective styling is a wonderful tool to help you achieve your long healthy hair goals.

Did You Know?

Twist outs and braids outs actually help to change your natural curl pattern, and braids or loose buns are good for protecting the hair while sleeping.

If you're thinking, "I am new to protective styling . . . where should I begin?" Once you get comfortable with the hair routine discussed in Chapter 1, begin perfecting certain styles throughout designated weeks. Now, your hair routine will look something like this: remember, routines train the hair to do what you want it to do on a weekly basis. Twist outs and braid outs are exceptional methods of protective styling that effectively protect the hair while simultaneously training the hair. Limited heat, incorporated training, increased protective styles, and proper cleansing are fantastic ways to kick-start your overall hair growth.

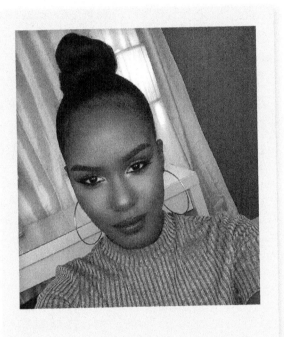

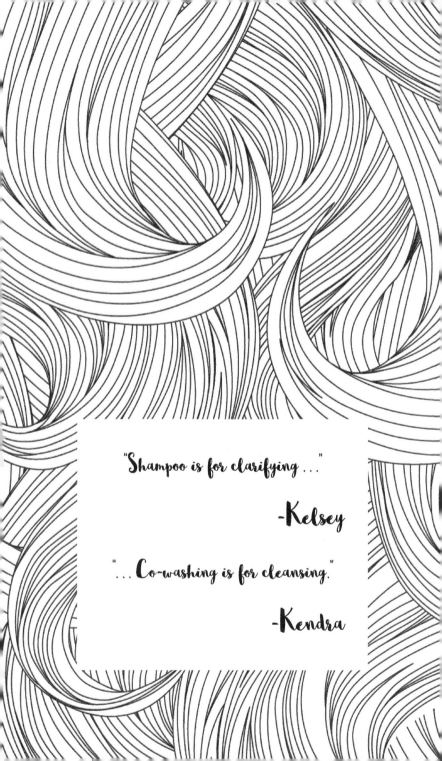

"Shampoo is for clarifying . . ."

-Kelsey

". . . Co-washing is for cleansing."

-Kendra

CHAPTER 3:
PROPER
SHAMPOOING

"Aaaahhhh," the ever-tempting sound of pleasure—that's what you hear from the amazingly gorgeous woman on the other side of the flat, translucent screen. The heightened sensation seems unquestionably overwhelming. The feeling is so overpowering and the smell so alluring, you notice her consciousness seems to momentarily escape her. She has never experienced anything so gratifying. "Yeeeessss!" Slowly, she runs her fingers through the white, thick substance, massaging her scalp ever so lightly. For the first time, she has experienced the climatic numbness one can only distinguish as the perfect shampoo!

We've all seen her. Laughably, every one, five, or seven days, you might just be her—that girl you see in the commercials shampooing with a head full of white soapy foam, cleansing her hair from tip to root. Unfortunately, her cleansing method is not the best or the healthiest.

Over time, advertising initiatives and marketing campaigns have sensationalized shampooing as a mandatory step for freshness, vitality, and luster. Nevertheless, while the outlandish image of that commercial shampoo is not an accurate reflection of the full physical effects of a great hair cleanser, it is typical of what most people do when washing their locks in the shower. Creating and massaging a head full of white suds is an accurate description of the method most people use to cleanse their strands.

So, why do you shampoo your hair? *"To clean it . . . duh"* (yeah, we predicted that response). That's not what we mean. After all, that is the simple answer—right? Cleaning your hair is probably not the only reason you shampoo. Take a moment and really consider *why* you shampoo? If you are honest, you likely shampoo regularly because you always have, because *they* said so, and because it has become habit. Unfortunately, if you shampoo the commercial way, it is probably a habit you should break.

Think About It

Of course shampooing can provide long-lasting benefits if done properly. Conversely, it can cause extreme detriments if done incorrectly. First, excessive shampooing can be incredibly damaging.

When you shampoo your hair too often, you are not giving your natural oils a chance to travel all the way to the ends of your hair. More notably, shampooing incorrectly on a daily or weekly basis can strip hair of its natural oils, making it dry and unhealthy.

For example, if your hair is bone straight, when your body secretes natural oils or you physically moisturize your strands, the moisture simply falls down the hair strand from root to tip. An effective moisturizing routine for the straight scenario is a simplistic task. In fact, it is often easy to over-moisturize straighter, thinner hair, causing a heavy residue or greasy appearance. On the other hand, if your hair is thick, curly, or coily, chances are you have a hard time maintaining moisture.

Maintaining moisture is more difficult for curly, burly hair because oils and moisture must travel a longer distance to moisturize from root to tip. When curly hair is moisturized, instead of a free-fall over a downward slope, it must travel around . . . and around . . . and around . . . and around . . . and around . . . and around . . . the curly loops of your locks. Hence, the road traveled is harder for moisture on the path of incredibly kinky curls. That is why your hair probably begins to look better the longer you maintain a style. Unfortunately, because mama instructed you to shampoo weekly or daily, as soon as your hair starts to look good, you strip all of its newly acquired moisture. Just as the moisture has found its way down your ravishing curls, you shampoo it again! Essentially, you have to start all over.

We all want longer, healthier hair right? (That's the point of this book). If length preservation is truly key, then you must understand that your hair requires constant moisture to eliminate breakage and decrease damage. Additionally, if you over-shampoo your hair regularly, it will be impossible to maintain moisture, and you will never be able to eliminate breakage. Shampooing incorrectly and too frequently can hinder the look and feel of those healthy strands, making the hair unappealingly dry and unusually brittle.

 Kelsey & Kendra's Confession

We too are guilty of the commercial poo. We have not always known the correct way to shampoo. For years, even during the beginning of our journey as vloggers, we would saturate our hair with water, fill our hands with a product of choice, and anticipate the soap-filled lather to which we had grown accustomed. We had never considered that our hair-cleansing methods were flawed. After all, you don't know what you don't know, because you don't know it.

What we did know was that after we washed our hair, it was always a tangled mess, and the innumerable knotted strands required an immense amount of time and effort. Then, on one remarkable day, our perception of hair cleansing changed. While we were watching YouTube videos on shampoo and conditioning routines, we came across one YouTuber in particular who asked, "So, why do you shampoo?"

She began explaining that while shampoo cleans all the "bad stuff" from your hair, it strips all of the good stuff too. It was as if a lightbulb went off. It simply made sense. We realized we lathered our hair weekly simply because our mom, grandma, and stylist said we should. We immediately began changing our hair-cleaning routine and saw instantaneous results. Our hair was undeniably softer, and we were able to cut our detangling time in half.

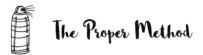 ## The Proper Method

"Lather, rinse, repeat" It's not a myth. In fact, this simple, three-step process is probably the most effective shampooing method.

We realized we did not necessarily have to "shampoo" to clean our hair. Ultimately, *sudsy* is not a synonym for *clean*. Although the commercial girls' sexy suds look appealing, they aren't required for cleanliness. Here's what you should know:

Shampoo Is Actually A Process For Your Roots—Not Your Strands.

When you are shampooing, wash your hair in sections. When you wash each section, only lather your roots. This method cleans the dirtiest part of the hair – the scalp. Focusing on your roots will diminish any build-up that can/will clog the pores at the onsite of the hair shaft. Also, when you shampoo the roots only, a smaller quantity of natural oils are removed from each hair strand, thereby increasing softness and decreasing tangles. We know this process may be cumbersome, but it's better than having tangles and breakage every time you wash.

If You Never Shampoo Your Hair Strands, You Would Still Maintain Clean, Healthy Hair.

Your newly focused attention on your root/scalp does not mean that you are neglecting the length of your hair strand. Don't worry, the rest of your tresses will get clean as you rinse the shampoo from the roots. Once the shampoo is applied to the hair, it's only point of exit during the rinse phase is down the hair strand. Hence, the length of each strand will receive cleaning by default.

When It Comes To Your Roots, Twice Is The Magic Number.

Though this is not a hard and fast rule, you will likely benefit from two scalp/root-shampoo-applications during each wash. As a general rule, the first wash eliminates unwanted dirt, excess oil, and product residue out of the hair. Conversely, the second wash actually cleanses the hair and does what the product is designed to do (i.e. moisturize, volumize, etc.).

Recognize The Alternatives.

Decreased shampoos does not mean dirtier hair. There are alternatives to shampoo that cleanse the hair without stripping its essentials. Shampoo substitutes include, but are not limited to: co-washing, sulfate-free shampoo, and dry shampoo.

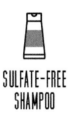

CO-WASHING

Co-washing is a poular cleansing method used by curly girls. Both conditioners and cleansing, conditioners are used to clean the hair without over drying it. The conditioner is applied to the hair in the place of shampoo. Although no large suds are formed, the hair is cleansed and its moisture is maintained.

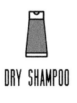

SULFATE-FREE SHAMPOO

Sulfate-free shampoos are cleansers that are free of sulfate. Sulfates are often found in household cleaners, like bathroom soaps and kitchen detergents which can be harmful to hair. First, sulfate-free shampoos are gentler. In addition, sulfate-free shampoos get the hair just as clean without stripping it of its natural oils. These shampoos are also the most universal shampoo for all hair types.

DRY SHAMPOO

Dry shampoos are sold in a dry powder spray form. They can temporarily clean the hair until wash day approaches. Dry shampoos are a life saver if you are trying to extend your styles.

Mix It Up & Write It Down.

Have you ever heard that if you take an over-the-counter medication too frequently eventually its effect on your symptoms may subside? Your hair is no different. After repeat use of certain products, your hair can become somewhat immune to the effect(s) of the product. That is why it is important that you alternate products periodically. While this is a crucial step, it requires a certain amount of accuracy and precision.

Do Not Change Products Too Frequently.

Use a product long enough to determine if it is one from which you may benefit; nonetheless, do not overuse the product either (do not determine a favorite product and develop an unwillingness to change it up.)

Once you change it up, write it down. This step will save you both time and money. For instance, if you try a product that leaves your hair feeling hard or dry, write down the product name and its ingredients. Maintain a journal of these products and periodically compare each entry. You may discover trends that you would not have otherwise determined. Perhaps it is the use of a particular ingredient to which your hair is resistant. You will learn to refrain from buying products that contain that ingredient. This method also works in the reverse, monitoring products that leave your hair feeling great. You may discover products that your hair tends to favor.

Shampooing Is Another Intricate Part Of Your Hair Routine.

We cannot say it enough: routines train the hair to do what you want it to do on a daily, weekly, and monthly basis. All hair reacts well to a routine. During your trial and error phase of your routine development, you will learn what feels good to your hair. Eventually, you will know how often to shampoo, how frequently to use an alternative, and what products to use more regularly.

Don't Get It Twisted

We are not suggesting that you stop washing your hair. Likewise, we would never advocate uncleanness. We are not even promoting the infamous "no-poo" method (a practice by which many women never use shampoo). Our two-part argument is simple:

(1) too much of a good thing can be detrimental, and
(2) improper use of a beneficial practice could become meaningless.

First, when it comes to shampoo, ask yourself, "*Why?*"
What is the point of that routine wash every 24-48 hours... bi-weekly... or monthly? Perhaps such a routine is necessary for your hair in particular. Chances are, nonetheless, that you have never really stopped to consider the why nor monitored the benefits of discontinuing your current wash schedule.

Second, even if you have mastered the timing aspects of your routine washes, there is a proper and improper method by which you can complete each wash. Your large lather is not proof of a better cleanser because the best cleanses do not always require lather.

What we are saying is natural oils coat the hair shaft and protect it while keeping it shiny and healthy. If you are constantly washing away those oils, you are stripping away that needed protection, desired luster, and preferred shine. What we are saying is to ignore the commercialized method of hair cleansing.

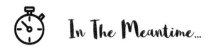 In The Meantime...

You will never know the possible effects of altering your hair cleansing method until you try it. Ignore that feeling of apprehension, and break the lather-filled monotony. Just try it out and see how your hair reacts to the changes you implement.

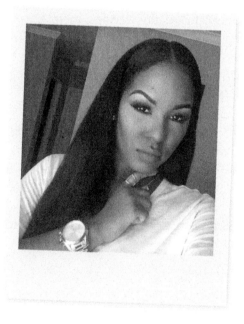

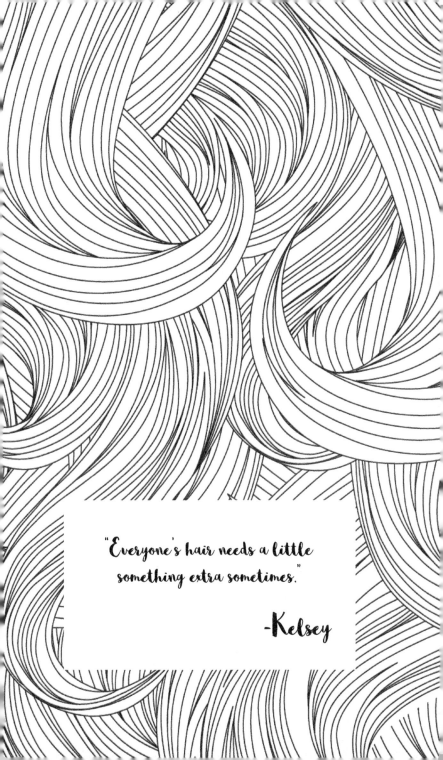

"Everyone's hair needs a little something extra sometimes."

-Kelsey

CHAPTER 4:
DEEP
CONDITIONING

Let's prepare a main course! Cooking this dish will be an unbelievably simple task. You will need a broiler and salt. To get started, fill the broiler with water and a hint of salt. Next, bring the water to a rapid boil. Last, add a pack of your favorite pasta. After just minutes, your dry grainy pasta will transform itself into a light, moist, flavorful dish that seems to pair well with just about any sauce or side. This meal is as easy as, "just add water."

Call it a unique comparison, but deep conditioning and pasta have much in common! Much like pasta, without moisture your hair becomes dry, brittle, and straw-like. Your hair depends on moisture to maximize volume, increase shine, and prevent breakage. Maintaining that moisture is just another key to maintaining your ends and ultimately, length.

Deep conditioning is to hair what water is to the body... what water is to the skin... what water is to most traditional Italian dishes... MOISTURE!! Much like increased water consumption provides numerous benefits to the body, regular *deep* conditioning treatments offer an unlimited number of benefits to the hair. Proper deep conditioning routines can mean improved overall health, strength, and volume. Nevertheless, a poor deep conditioning routine (or failure to deep condition), may have horrific results. Brace yourself, because failure to maintain moisture likely means a broom-like appearance or dry-pasta-like result.

Think About It

When you add pasta to a pot of rapidly boiling water, the pasta swells, causing all of the grain consistency to move to the surface of the pasta. Its starches run out so it can conceal moisture within. Eventually, the noodles' starches are boiled into the water, removing its brittle texture, trapping the moisture inside, and revealing a soft, succulent, lustrous result.

Your hair is no different. When you deep condition, you not only moisturize your hair, but you allow the hair an opportunity to trap the added moisture. The additional moisture increases buoyancy, softness, shine, and STREGNTH. While we would never recommend boiling your hair, as you'll learn later in this chapter, for a penetrating deep conditioner a disposable shower cap coupled with low heat has much the same effect as boiling pasta.

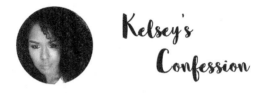

I have also experienced some heat damage. Although I have never experienced the level of heat damage as Kendra discusses in Chapter One, I have struggled to maintain my natural curls from root to tip. Even from my early days of transitioning, I would always find that after winter straightening, I would lose the tip end of my curl pattern. It took me a while to love my naturally curly hair because even after the transition was complete, I still had a lot of straight pieces that were heat damaged. After a good cleansing, I was left with a head full of beautiful curls and a few strands of straight ends. Of course, I could have just cut them off, but I did not want to give up on the length. No matter what product I used, those straight ends refused to curl.

Nevertheless, I was determined to save the hair or at minimum, the length those ends provided.

At the time, I was new to the world of non-processed hair, and had no knowledge of the benefits of deep conditioning. But I knew that heat damage often lead to dry, brittle, moisture-resistant hair. I also knew that I ran the risk of those dry, brittle, moisture-resistant ends splitting up my hair shaft. I figured if I could keep the ends moisturized, I could prevent the splitting and maintain moisture long enough to grow my hair from the root as I slowly trimmed and removed the ends. The only problem was no product seemed to help me maintain moisture from co-wash to co-wash. Then, I found deep conditioning!

Implementing a deep conditioning routine totally repaired my hair. The first time I deep conditioned, I could not believe how soft and bouncy my hair was. Also, I immediately noticed my hair was stronger. A few of those ends even produced a small loop or half curl (lol!), which made the heat damage less noticeable. I was so happy with the results, for about two months, I began deep conditioning every three days. Surprisingly, my full curls slowly bounced back. Deep conditioning salvaged my ends and saved my length. I was ecstatic, and I was hooked. After seeing the benefits of deep condition, Kendra began implementing deep conditioning into her hair routine as well. Still, today, we consider a good deep conditioner the most critical part of our hair routine.

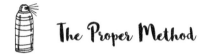

The Proper Method

What is the Difference between Conditioner and Deep Conditioner?

It is no secret that dry unconditioned hair can cause breakage up the hair shaft. That is why maintaining moisture while transitioning is so crucial. Unfortunately, substituting a deep conditioner with the regular conditioner that comes with matching shampoo is often, on its own, not as effective. Conditioners and deep conditioners provide two separate aspects of conditioning and moisture provision. Here are just a few of the differences:

SIMPLE CONDITIONER

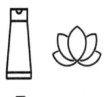

- ◊ Makes hair softer
- ◊ Bottle reads, *conditioner*
- ◊ Leave in for two-three minutes as instructed
- ◊ No heat necessary
- ◊ Short-term results
- ◊ Often comes in a bottle

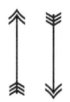

DEEP CONDITIONER

- ◊ Makes hair shinier, less dense, and stronger
- ◊ Bottle reads, *deep conditoner or hair mask*
- ◊ Leave in for ten to 30 minutes as instructed
- ◊ Low, indirect heat suggested
- ◊ Long-term results
- ◊ Likely comes in a jar

The paired conditioner lacks ingredients for penetration into the hair shaft. While the product paired conditioner is good, it only preps the hair for deep conditioning. Just consider the regular conditioner as the pre-show and the deep conditioner as the "main event."

Did You Know?

Adding any natural oil, like coconut oil, to conditioner can alter its quality, making it more like deep conditioner. This is an acceptable substitute if you run out product. Still, do not make it a regular practice. After all, there ain't nothing like the real thing!

What Type of Deep Conditioner Should I Use?

Deep conditioner can achieve many types of results. The paper label on your product of choice will reveal the conditioner "type" or intended result. For instance, it may read "moisturizing deep conditioning treatment" or "strengthening hair mask." Because all hair needs moisture, anything with the word, "moisture," on it is universal. However, if your hair is breaking off and is on the weaker side, try a strengthening deep conditioner. If you need both moisture and strength, find a product that has both qualities. Also, if you are having problems with frizz, smoothing deep conditioners are the way to go. The bottom line is, the type of deep conditioner you use depends on what your hair needs. No matter the type of deep conditioner you select, deep conditioning is one of the best things you can do for your hair.

How Do I Deep Condition?

In addition to purchasing the proper product, you must utilize the proper application process.

First, do not put deep conditioner on the root of your hair. Remember deep conditioning is used to revitalize the hair and replenish moisture. The bottom part of the hair is the oldest. The hair closest to your roots is the newest hair and likely will not need additional moisture because your hair cuticle secretes natural oils. The hair that has grown out, the farthest away from the root probably lacks moisture because the naturally secreted moisture must travel so far down the hair shaft (for a better explanation, see Chapter 2).

Technically, adding moisture to your root voids your shampoo. In Chapter 4, we suggest shampooing the roots and allowing your rinse to cleanse the oldest parts of the hair. Here we are merely suggesting the opposite. If you add the deep conditioner at the root, you are inadvertently replacing the excess oil you just removed from the scalp. So, adding moisture at the root or the portion of the strand close to the root will result in overly-oily hair, giving the hair a limp, heavy, volumeless appearance. Instead, focus on the second half of your length, avoiding the roots and scalp. Try applying your product of choice from the ears downward. This will create a balance of moisture (natural oils at the root and added moisture at the ends).

After the product is applied, allow it to remain in the hair for the suggested amount of time which will be anywhere from ten to 30 minutes. For the best results, put on a disposable shower cap and sit under a dryer with low heat while you wait. The extra step creates a penetrating deep conditioner. If you choose not to sit under a dryer just leave it on for 30 minutes to an hour for the same results. Much like the boiling water increases moisture absorption ability for pasta, a low level of heat will improve moisture retention for your hair. The heat opens the hair shaft, increasing absorption to the third power, helping each strand trap the maximum amount of applied moisture. The cap acts as a protective cover, allowing your hair to reap the benefits of the increased temperature without direct heat.

What is the Most Common Deep Conditioning Mistake?

Beyond applying the deep conditioning treatment to the entire hair stand, another common mistake is what we call ponytail application. You are probably familiar with this practice. This is when you squeeze product in your hands, rub them together, and gather all of your hair as if to style a ponytail. All of your hair is gathered in one or both hands. You apply the product root to tip, completely saturating the hair on the outside of the pony tail, moving your pony hold from the scalp to the end of the hair. The problem is, more than just the perimeter of the hair needs deep conditioning. This application method neglects the hair inside the pony. To avoid this issue, do not apply product to your hair in a ponytail fashion; instead, gently finger rake the product through the hair. Doing so will minimize breakage in the center.

How Often Should I Deep Condition?

Regular deep conditioning will be different for every person. An average routine includes weekly or bi-weekly deep conditioning. However, variances reflect the individualized needs of your hair. We suggest no more than once per week, but no less than one application every two weeks—unless your hair demands more or less. What we mean is it all depends on the overall health of your hair and your regular hair routine. During the healing stage of Kelsey's Confession, she deep conditioned once every 72-hours. Whether it be once a week or once every two weeks, both are good time frames. Just listen to your hair. When you implement deep conditioner, you will notice the difference in texture, feel, and appearance. When your hair begins to feel overly-dry, try deep conditioning again. You may find the proceeding deep conditioner to be just as effective. If so, maintain that time frame. If you dislike the results or see no results at all, elongate the time between the ineffective deep conditioning treatment and the one that you should follow. Do not worry, you will get in your groove and fall in love with your hair.

We do firmly suggest, however, that you monitor how often you use the same product for deep conditioning treatments. If you are like us, you will develop a favorite deep conditioning mask, but avoid using it for every deep conditioning treatment. Using the same product repeatedly will cause your hair to build immunities to the product, and each application will become less effective. So, change it up every couple of months or rotate your products of choice.

Don't Go Cheap!

Better products may be more expensive. If you are used to only buying a shampoo and conditioner pair, the price difference between conditioner and a deep conditioning cream may be a bit of a shock. For instance, though our favorite deep conditioners range from $15 to $40, we have spent up to $50 on a jar of deep conditioner. We have learned better products are more expensive for a reason. Often, they have a thicker consistency, requiring less product during each application. Hence, the jar lasts longer and you break even!

Don't Get It Twisted

We are not suggesting you drive to the nearest salon or closest store and buy the most expensive product on the shelf. We will be disappointed if you inbox us reporting your first $100 product purchase with no supporting explanation as to why you selected the product or what benefits you anticipated. We are simply saying do your research. Look at product reviews and ingredients. Try to avoid letting the price guide your pick. Instead, let the product determine your selection. The benefit of the product should be primary, and the price should be secondary. Consider it an investment into your long-term hair goals.

You will never know the possible effects of altering your hair cleansing method until you try it, fail or succeed, and try again. It is a process. Enjoy the ride and ignore the feelings of apprehension. Just try it out, and see how your hair reacts to the changes you implement.

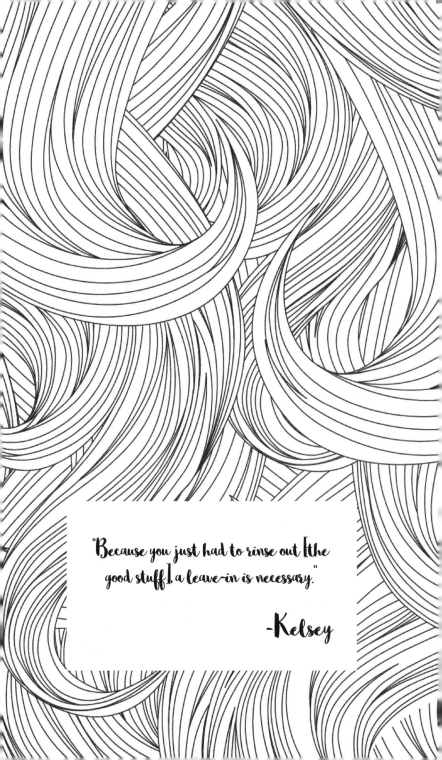

"Because you just had to rinse out [the good stuff], a leave-in is necessary."

-Kelsey

CHAPTER 5:
LEAVE-IN CONDITIONERS

"Baby, you look like you took a bath in flour, and I know we didn't bake cakes today. Go in the house and put on some lotion!" That is what you'd hear my grandmother say if you attempted to leave her house without moisturizing your skin. She understood that moisturizing the skin regularly increases elasticity, disallows wrinkles, and prevents cracking of the skin. Plus, as she so eloquently put it (lol!), lubricant application just looks better.

You need a good wash, rinse, and lubricant to maintain healthy-looking skin. If you regularly skip any of these steps, the formula is broken and you are at risk for premature dryness, breaking, wrinkles, and any other adverse effects of not using a lubricant.

Leave-in conditioners are to the hair what lotions are to the skin. Once lotions and leave-in conditioners are applied, your hair and skin just look better. Leave-ins are equivalent to applying lotion after the shower. You can—but it is best not to skip this step. Leave-ins give the hair the perfect amount of moisture and manageability before styling.

Think About It

Alright, we get it. First, we just told you to lose the heat; then, we told you to change your wash and conditioning routine, incorporate a deep conditioning routine, and now we are suggesting you implement a leave-in conditioner routine. You are probably thinking, "Do I really need all of that?" Yes, you do! It is easy to believe that if you just skip one of these steps it is *not that big of a deal*. However, over time, it can become a big deal. It could mean the difference in maintaining an extra three or five inches this year.

Plus, why not? Why shouldn't you complete all of these steps? You do the "steps" for every other part of your body from big to small. For instance, when you manicure your nails (if you are doing it properly) you clip, file, clean, and dry. Then, you apply a base coat, two color coats, and a top coat. Experimental painting will quickly prove that if you skip any of these steps the final product just doesn't look the same.

For another example, when you brush your teeth you floss, brush, and rinse. Then, you use a mouthwash, tongue scrapper, and may even use a whitening treatment. Dental maintenance requires many steps, but you do not skip steps, because skipping leads to cavities, bad breath, and stains.

Furthermore, during your nighttime routine, you use a makeup remover. Then, you wash your face, rinse accordingly, apply a toner, and moisturize. Multiple instances of step skipping will only lead to red spots, blackheads, and breakouts. We could go on and on. The point is, as women, we rarely skip steps except when it comes to our hair. Why? Likely because each step can be costly and it is more time consuming than any of the steps involved in nail care, skin maintenance, and dental upkeep. Also, many women are accustomed to going to the salon twice a month, which may be infrequent but necessary. Your hair may require weekly maintenance and that every-other-week trip to the stylist may not be enough to get the results you desire. Moreover, going to the salon is not a substitute or excuse for failure to regularly maintenance your own hair or to recognizing when in-between care is needed.

Leave-in conditioners are more of a moisturizing styling product than a cleansing product. Perhaps that is why many people think that leave-in conditioners are optional in their hair routines. This is another nasty hair fallacy. Leave-in application is a grossly important step. In fact, leave-in conditioners should be considered more mandatory than other stylers. Hairspray, gels, and serums are regular stylers, but are optional. However, leave-in conditioners are very mandatory.

Why Leave-Ins?

Unlike cream conditioners and deep conditioners, leave-ins are light. Think of cream conditioners and deep fried chicken. The chicken is succulent and moist, but not too healthy. Now imagine leave-in conditioners as oven-fried chicken (if you have ever had it). It gives you the crunch of oil-fried chicken without the heaviness.

Simply put, leave-in conditioners are essential for hair integrity. Leave-ins are saviors, salvaging and prepping your strands for heat application from blow-dryers, and curling irons, and flat irons. Second, leave-ins can act as a detangler, preventing the need to use harsh finger detangling remedies. Lastly, leave-ins have the potential to sooth the hair, preventing curl knots and fairy knots. All of these can be detrimental to the hair, causing breakage and prolonging your healthy hair goals.

Are You Having Trouble Maintaining Your Style?

Additionally, when we use leave-ins we notice our hair is even softer and bouncier and our styling lasts longer. If your hair frizzes easily or you find that your styles are not long-lasting, you should invest in a good leave-in conditioner. Style-maintenance is a collateral benefit to leave-ins. Because they create a smoothing barrier around the hair, they inadvertently cause your hairs to stay in place for longer periods of time.

What Type of Leave-In Conditioner Should I Use?

Of course, you should use the leave-ins that provide the best results for your hair or leave-ins that are suggested for your hair type. Leave-ins generally comes in two forms, a spray form or a creamy/liquid foam. As licensed cosmetologists we have noticed that creamy/liquid leave-ins work best for our clients with thicker, coarser hair. On the other hand, (you guessed it), as a general rule, if your hair is on the finer, thinner side, then a spray form is likely better. For thinner, straighter hair, spray conditioners provide a lighter feel. This will prevent the look of oily weighted hair.

When you are looking for a good leave-in conditioner, there are some benefits you should look for. Search the aisle for leave-in conditioners that read: "protects against heat," "eliminates frizz," or "improve elasticity and minimizes breakage." Find the leave-in that promises results that are solutions to any difficulties you may be experiencing with your hair. Basically, match the description with your needs.

How Do I Apply Leave-In Conditioners

First, we recommended that you apply your leave-ins to damp hair after your deep conditioning treatment has been rinsed out thoroughly. Remember, damp hair creates more opportunity for product penetration. Furthermore, if you are at the point in your hair routine where you are implementing heat, you will be glad to learn that heat styling, like blow drying seals and soothes hair in which leave-in conditioner has been applied. (This is another collateral affect that gives your style(s) frizz-free longevity). Then, use your leave-in of choice in conjunction with a wide-tooth comb, paddle brush, or detangler of choice.

WARNING: If you prefer a paddle brush while detangling, brush the product through in a vertical rather than a horizontal motion.

Adding your leave-in conditioner should always be the very first step before styling. After today, think of leave-in conditioners as the ultimate styling product. They offer double the benefits, sealing, smoothing, and protecting the hair while creating a long-lasting, frizz-free style. Even if you choose not to apply any other styling products, you now know a leave-in conditioner is a must-have to maintaining healthy hair and helping you reach your healthy hair goals.

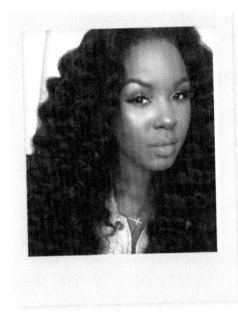

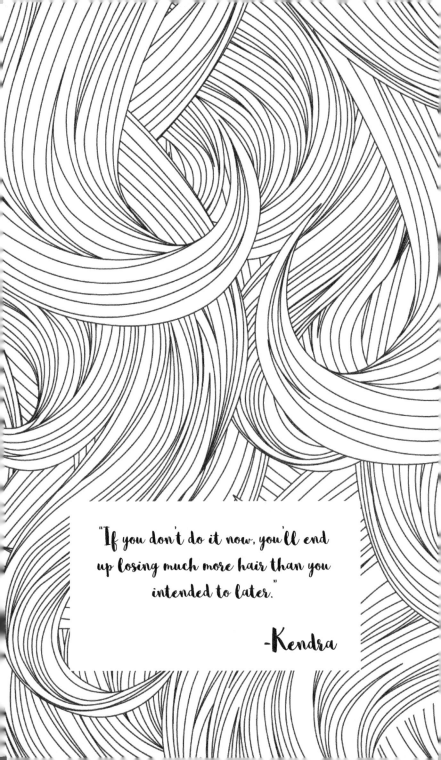

"If you don't do it now, you'll end up losing much more hair than you intended to later."

-Kendra

CHAPTER 6:
TRIMMING

Yes, this is a book about growing longer, healthier hair . . . and yes, we are telling you that in order to grow long hair YOU NEED A TRIM. Trimming can be the most dreaded part of hair maintenance. Of course, very few clients will call a professional stylist excited about trimming their locks. Instead, they call and request some other service like a wash and deep conditioning treatment. However, on the day of the appointment, during the entire drive, they pray that the stylist does not say those dreaded words: "Your ends need trimming."

As professional stylists, we understand both ends of the spectrum. As the one in need of a trim, Kelsey vowed not to lose all of her split ends at once during her transition phase. Her decision, however, was accompanied by many risks. By cutting only a portion of her split ends at a time, she ran the risk of the split moving rapidly up her hair shaft. To combat the risk, as mentioned in Chapter 4, she deep conditioned every two or three days. Her choice was not only risky, but also time consuming and expensive.

On the other hand, as professional stylists, we also know the feeling of delivering that dreaded news. The client (who subconsciously knows she is in need of a trim), sits nervously in the chair as her bun is loosened or her hat is removed. Through her peripheral vision, she gazes through her stylist's station wall mirror. As the stylist begins to examine her hair and intensely focuses specifically on her ends, her mood shifts from subtle nervousness to overwhelming concern. Her face tightens and her palms begin to sweat. Then, the stylist meets her gaze in the mirror and smiles.

We have seen it too many times. Repeatedly, we have had to speak those dreaded words: "Your ends need trimming." It is generally an awkward moment, and more often than not, the expression on the client's face screams, "Say it ain't so . . . say it ain't so!" Sound familiar?

When you work tirelessly to grow your hair, it is natural to feel cheated when some of that length has to be removed. However, instead of feeling like your hard work is falling to the floor, cheer up. The truth of the matter is trimming your hair is a good thing. The process of cutting dead, frizzy, frazzled ends enables you to maintain additional length more quickly over time.

The bottom line is, if you want to grow long, healthy hair trimming should never be avoided.

Ever snagged a fingernail or gotten a hang nail? Both can be annoying and painful. For instance, the dreaded snagged nail always rears its head a day or two before a scheduled nail appointment. When it occurs, what's a normal, natural reaction? Preserve the length of that nail. In an attempt to make sure the nail will last until your appointment, you get creative. Our favorite methods is the clear polish mending technique. You try to polish the pieces of the nail together hoping it will be enough to mend it for 48 hours. We have all tried it. It only takes a few failed attempts to learn that as long as the nail is snagged, it will get caught in any and everything, continuously ripping across the nail bed until the entire nail is lost. It takes very few attempts to realize that the best way to preserve the nail is to file or cut out the snag, creating a straight, smooth corner of the nail.

The same is true for hang nails. When that small flap of skin starts to peel down your finger, it is painful. The pain, however, is worsened following failure to cut out the hanging skin. The skin will continue to split down your finger until it eventually begins to bleed. Thankfully, just one small snip from the nail clippers prevents approaching pain, eliminates further splitting, and enables abrupt healing. The splitting skin and nail is much like splitting hair.

If left untrimmed, split ends will travel up the length of your hair, inadvertently causing perfectly good layers of your locks to become brittle and damaged. Avoiding much needed trims will almost always make matters worse. This is because split ends are not repairable. Eventually, your hair will become so damaged that you will have to cut your hair instead of trimming the ends. Simply put, trimming your ends should be a happy moment, because the sooner you rid your hair of those damaged, frazzled ends, the less hair you have to cut off over time.

A Confidential Confession

I have been watching Kelsey and Kendra since the beginning of time – literally. Before they were professional stylists, fashion experts, or YouTube phenomenas, they were simply family. As two of my closest family members, I have had the opportunity to watch their hair care regimens from start to finish, and their "Get Ready with Me" uploads are literally an in-person experience for me.

My favorite time to watch (and ultimately mimic) their hair care routine, is during their curly months. During those months, when the girls prep their hair, I follow along and style my own. During one peculiar experience, I watched as Kelsey removed her silk bonnet, undoing her nightly pineapple and allowing her long curls to cascade down her back. Afterward, she sectioned the hair and used a spray bottle to moisten the curls. Then, I noticed that she began lifting the tips of her hair carefully examining the ends. She paused, opened a drawer and pulled out a bag. She began frivolously looking in the bag and retrieved a pair of shiny shears. Then, she quickly commenced the process of examining her ends. Next she separated a few ends, rubbed her fingers down her hair, and picked up the shears. It was at this moment that I realized her true intention. Before I could motion my mouth to speak, she began to snip about an inch of the curl. After its fall to the floor, I jolted across the bathroom screaming, "Noooooooo!!!! Are you crazy?" I asked. "Do you know how long it would take me to grow what you just cut off?"

Instead of answering my series of questions. Kelsey began laughing hysterically. I imagined what I must have looked like. I mentally played the scene back in slow motion. I looked like a crazed mad woman from a motion picture on a mission to prevent some prized possession from shattering across the floor as it fell. I began to laugh too.

Then, Kelsey explained the importance of trimming regularly. She said that a quest to keep split ends would always be uneventful and could actually result in a decrease in length. The idea actually made sense. I have always understood that my hair is constantly growing. Even during my relaxer days, it did not take a genius to realize the only reason there is ever a need for a touch up or retouch is because new growth has appeared. Still, despite my constant new growth and continuous need for a retouch, my hair was always shoulder length.

The trims were my missing piece. I rarely trimmed my ends. Perhaps my ends were splitting faster (or at least at the same rate) than my hair was growing. I implemented her advice immediately. Although I have never been bold enough to snip a split end on-site, I did begin getting trims as needed and on a regular basis. Following my big chop (which was boy cut short), I was able to grow a full second head of shoulder length hair in just a year's time.

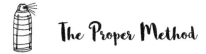

The Proper Method

Most women hate trims because they share the same unfortunate experience—some previous scissor happy stylist. They went to the salon in need of a trim and came out with a full haircut. The fear is understandable. People stay away from the salon simply for that reason. There are only two logical solutions.

First, learn to properly trim your own hair. Second, find a stylist that you trust. For most women, the first solution is not a viable option. If you are afraid to clip your ends or sacrifice the hair you will lose during the learning process, do not pressure yourself. For you, the biggest piece of hair-trimming advice we can offer is to find a good stylist. Have a conversation with that professional, share your hair goals, and be upfront about past unfavorable experiences. In addition, always remember, the worst that can happen is that the stylist cut an inch when you thought she should only cut a half inch. But, you know what? It is just hair, and for most of us God provides a never-ending supply. It will grow back, and with the proper hair routine it will grow back healthier, thicker, stronger, and longer.

Our Trimming Routine

Our trimming routine has always been pretty simple. Since we started following the exact same steps in this book, we have found that following a stringent haircare routine and embracing trims when necessary has helped us retain length. Although we needed more frequent trims when we began this journey, now we usually only trim our hair twice a year. Yes, two trims per year is a realistic and obtainable goal.

We trim once before the summer just before we go curly. Then, we trim once in the fall or winter when we implement a straightening routine. The more you embrace the need to trim, the less you will actually need them; the healthier your hair becomes, the fewer split ends you will find, and the less frequent your trips to the trimming chair will become.

How Often Should I Get Trims?

The frequency of your trims will totally depends on your individual needs. While the overall health of your hair is a major factor, your choice of style will also play a part in your trimming regimen. For instance, shorter cuts require more maintenance, while longer hair generally demands fewer trims each year.

Learn to listen to your hair. Your hair's ability to perform or not perform as usual are clues that your hair is in need of something. For instance, if you can easily create and maintain voluminous curls and all of a sudden your hair isn't holding a curl it's probably because you need a trim. Likewise, if you can usually detangle easily and detangling or combing becomes a hassle you are likely in need of a trim. You will always get better results and your hair will be easier to maintain with trimmed ends.

How To Recognize Split Ends

Detecting split ends is an easy task. Once you know what a split end looks like, recognizing them is as easy as *letters and limbs*. When your hair is down or in a neatly style ponytail, divide the hair into small sections. Then, taking the ends of each section between two fingers, examine the tips or ends of the strands in that particular section. Next, visually identify and survey the individual strands. A healthy strand of hair begins and ends as one single strand of hair. If a single piece of hair is smooth and then becomes a Y before the end of the strand, it is split. However, a Y is only one of many types of splits. Splits may appear as two or more Z's or multiple splits, much like tree limbs.

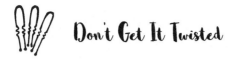 # Don't Get It Twisted

We are not recommending a trim every time you visit the salon. What we are suggesting is learning when trims are necessary. Doing so is a process that becomes easier with an established hair routine. A regular haircare regimen will help you better understand your hair and its needs. While Girl A may need a trim bi-monthly, Girl B may only require a trim bi-annually.

More importantly, we are not endorsing self-help as the solution to split ends for every girl. Kelsey's find 'em and clip 'em routine may not be the best option for you. Remember, we have the benefit of being card-carrying, certified cosmetologists. Furthermore, we have each other. So, when one of us needs a trim the other is always available to provide the service or mend any self-inflicted cutting fiascos. For women who choose not to self-clip, what we are stressing is the importance of deciding who you can trust to trim your ends.

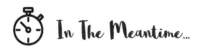 In The Meantime...

Trims are a necessary component to truly growing and maintaining longer, healthier hair. Whether you take the time to self-trim or you seek a professional cut, trimming must be done. For the latter, find a stylist who knows how to treat your texture/grade of hair and understands the difference between a haircut and trim. Whichever you chose, do not make excuses in an attempt to avoid an inevitable trim. We promise, if you cut the lifeless, frail parts now, you will be able to sit back and watch the thriving parts of your hair grow beautifully later.

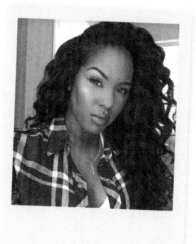

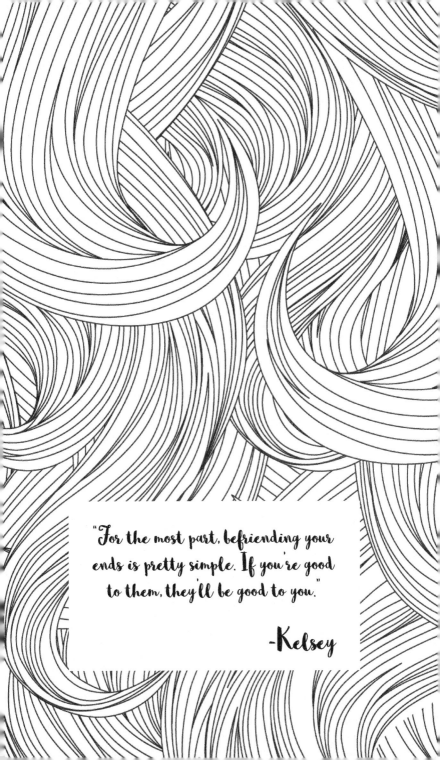

"For the most part, befriending your ends is pretty simple. If you're good to them, they'll be good to you."

-Kelsey

CHAPTER 7:
BECOMING
FRIENDS WITH
YOUR ENDS

Kate was elated to receive flowers from Darrel. They had only been dating a week. He was so thoughtful, and the lilies he selected were beautiful. Of course, Kate clipped the stems and placed the bouquet in a crystal vase. She tried her best to water them, but they soon began to droop. She could not understand why a few of the petals turned brown after she added additional water. Then, she realized that perhaps the flowers were not getting enough sunlight. In an attempt to reverse her watering process, she sat the bouquet in the window sill. Still, Kate's lilies were lifeless. When she returned home from work, many of the petals and leaves were brown and others had fallen off the flowers. No matter what she tried, nothing worked. Apparently, there was no bringing this plant back to life. Finally, she trashed the flowers that she had been so happy to receive less than a week earlier.

Much like your hair, Kate's lilies require a delicate balance of ingredients and care to achieve and maintain life and luster. Kate was unsuccessful in sustaining her flowers because she failed to provide her flowers with soil, food, water, and sunlight. While each of these nutrients is required, too much of any one can be detrimental to overall growth. Your hair needs cleansing, conditioning, trimming, and moisturizing, but too much of any of these minimizes the balance that your hair requires. For instance, too much shampoo may lead to drying, which leads to brittleness and causes breakage.

Here is the thing: Your hair is always growing. Yes, unless you are battling alopecia or some other type of scalp disease, your hair is growing. So why are you not maintaining length? It is likely because your hair is breaking. Even healthy hair can break easily. You likely have some length of hair you grow easily. Then, the growth simply stops. However, the growth from your scalp has not stopped. It makes sense then that the length from the bottom of the strand has simply broken off.

Let's Recap

We have talked extensively about trimming and protecting your ends. Both are crucial steps in the quest for long, healthy hair. However, we want to be clear that this chapter is not a repeat of any of the prior chapters with ends-specific instructions. Remember our example about the hair-down-girl in Chapter 2? By the day's end, her hair had been brushed, combed, curled, straightened, pulled, buttoned, zipped, covered, blown, scrubbed, rubbed, curled, twirled, and rained on. Her behavior was detrimental to length retention, and she needed to work harder to protect her ends. We suggested buns, braids, and twists as a solution to protect your ends.

Next, in Chapter 6, we made a big deal about trimming your ends. Do you recall our hangnail analogy? We discussed how the small flap of skin will continuously peel until it is trimmed, and how one small snip from the nail clippers will eliminate further splitting and enable abrupt healing. Moreover, we warned that just like the hangnail, failure to trim split ends will cause further splitting. In that chapter, we focused on how to repair damaged hair by removing split ends.

In this chapter, the focus is unique. Once you implement all of the prior steps in this guide, you will start to achieve growth beyond the length to which you are accustomed. When your hair starts to respond and your locks grow, it is equally important to maintain your new, healthy ends. This chapter focuses on maintaining healthy ends once your hair is trained and repaired, and creating and maintaining a sort of life-long friendship with your ends.

Any length beyond your "natural length" is simply a length at which your hair is the most delicate. This is the length where your scalp has a more difficult time providing moisture to the end of the strand. Growing your hair to this length is easy, but getting growth beyond this length is difficult. Longer hair may experience additional pulling, zipping, rubbing, and combing. This is likely why you have to learn to provide your hair with the extra care and time it needs. This is why you must learn, through your personalized hair routine, when your ends need trimming, and it is also why protecting your ends with buns and braids is crucial. You must learn a new routine for this new length of hair.

To grow, a plant requires water, sunlight, and soil. Imagine a waterless plant. The roots are left dehydrated and the leaves become dry and brittle. Naturally, the plant dies. If attached to the root, nevertheless, the plant can often be repaired. However, to repair the plant, you will have to cut the dead leaves and replenish it with all three essential nutrients. As for the leaves, there is no saving them. Much like split ends, you must trim them and wait for the new, healthy hair to grow again. To avoid this vicious cycle of growth, breakage, and repair of split and dead ends, you must become friends with your ends. Improving the manner in which you care for your ends will not only allow you to maintain your current length, but it will also enable you to watch added length sprout from your roots. Retaining length through maintaining your ends is the only way you will see results.

Perhaps you are not seeing your desired length because you are not taking the necessary steps to care for the hair you already have. Hence, if your hair is damaged today and you implement all of the training from this book, your newly grown roots will appear healthier and stronger—and eventually, those new roots will become your well-maintained ends. Once this happens, you must take extra steps to ensure that those ends remain healthy and strong to avoid having to start this entire process again.

Becoming Friends With Your Ends

This is probably the easiest chapter of our guide to implement in your daily routine. The following steps are simple, every-day things you can do to better maintain your ends:

1. Keep your ends moisturized

Water is to plants as moisture is to hair. Beyond excessive heat, failing to moisturize those ends, is yet another way you might end up with cactus-like, dry, or prickly hair. That much-needed moisture is all around you. Moisturizers come in many forms. Consider one or any combination of conditioners, oils, and serums.

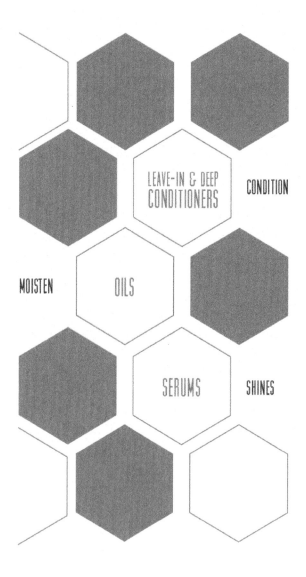

LEAVE-IN & DEEP
CONDITIONERS

CONDITION

MOISTEN

OILS

SERUMS

SHINES

 92

2. Don't leave your ends out while you are sleeping

Believe it or not, sleeping on your hair can be incredibly hazardous to hair growth—especially if you sleep on cotton sheets and pillowcases. Cotton is an oil-stripper. It absorbs moisture. As a result, after you have used your choice of a conditioner, oil, or serum and you hop in bed, the sheets will make better use of your oil application than your hair. Sleeping on loose hair may also be the reason you may be unable to maintain moisture.

To avoid depleting the moisture from your hair, refrain from leaving your locks loose when you sleep. Instead, try sleeping on a satin or silk pillowcase. Furthermore, instead of leaving your hair or ends out, try wrapping your hair with a silk scarf, putting it in a bun, or creating a braid. Changing something as small as your sleeping pattern will make a big difference in moisture retention, shine, and overall growth.

3. Avoid leaning or lying on your hair

Get off your hair! It is so delicate, and you should treat it as such. Even the strongest strand of hair is still a strand of hair. It can only take so much weight or stand so much pressure before it snaps. Lying on, sitting on, and tugging at your locks will weaken them. Unfortunately, when the hair is weak, the first part of the hair to break is its end. Sure, one broken end will not make a big difference, but another, after another, after another will quickly become noticeable. Then you will find yourself trimming dead ends or cutting uneven layers. So, if that end breaks, there will be a break in your overall growth retention.

Of course, many of us don't even notice when we aren't being delicate with our hair. We likely don't consider our locks during a long car ride or a quick nap. Nevertheless, often times lying or leaning on your hair can cause breakage, snagging, and drying.

Where It All Comes 2Gether

Each of these tips provides what is necessary to create that balance of nutrients you need to maintaining length. Developing the friendship between you and your ends may take some time, but if you put in the time and get to know your new BFF, you will experience unbelievable growth.

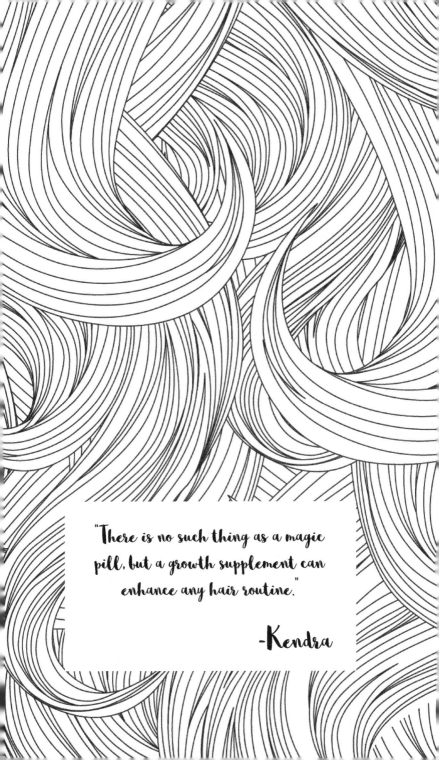

"There is no such thing as a magic
pill, but a growth supplement can
enhance any hair routine."

-Kendra

CHAPTER 8:
TAKING
SUPPLEMENTS

During Kim's lifestyle change, she was determined to lose 20 pounds, and she was confident that her freshly purchased bottle of weight loss pills would help her achieve her goal. During the first two weeks, she took her magic pill at the same time every day, just as the bottle's label instructed. Sadly, when Kim stepped on the scale, she learned that she had not lost weight. In fact, she gained a half a pound. The next week, Kim tried something new. In addition to taking the weight loss supplement, she exercised regularly, and implemented a clean eating schedule. Within three weeks, she lost nearly ten pounds.

After reading the title of this chapter, we are sure your heart began beating faster, your adrenaline started running quicker, your eyes widened, and your lips turned upward. If you thought to yourself, "Yeeeesss honey, they are about to tell me which pill they used to make their hair 24 inches long," perhaps your excitement grew from an unrealistic expectation.

"Is there is a magic pill to make my hair grow?" is probably one of the most frequently asked questions we get from subscribers on our YouTube channels, GlamTwinz334 and GlamTwinzTV. The answer is, "not exactly." Our hair did not descend from the confines of some plastic bottle, and yours will not either. However, do not be discouraged. When used properly, supplements can enhance hair growth and decrease overall wait time for growth. The key is correctly implementing the proper supplement in your hair routine.

Think About It

If you are taking a supplement and doing nothing else, even if your hair grows longer faster the result will be short-lived. Even if your hair grew 10 times faster and you failed to protect your hair, moisturize your locks, and condition your strands, you would not see the length that would result from the new growth. Your hair would grow faster, demanding more care, moisture, trimming, and oil. In the event that you did not improve these areas of care, the hair would break anyway. If you have yet to develop a routine with which you are providing your hair with those key things today, an influx of growth will just become more problematic tomorrow.

Kim experienced the best results when she began a regular workout routine coupled with a proper diet and weight loss supplement. The same holds true for hair vitamins. Supplements are very helpful in the hair growth process, but they are not your saving grace. Many people take supplements, thinking the daily capsules will do all the work they should be doing. WRONG! You still have to put in work.

A carefully selected hair growth supplement is an internal way to speed up your hair growth process. However, contrary to popular belief, there is no pill guaranteed to take you from ten to twenty inches in a month. Hair growth will never happen that way.

Supplement Benefits

Most people use supplements to reach a longer length of hair. Still, many users do not know that supplements improve more than just growth—they can help with the overall health of the hair. This may include, thicker locks and less breakage, among other things. The following list provides many of the benefits your hair vitamin(s) may provide:

- Increasing luster/shine
- Improving strength
- Providing elasticity
- Preventing hair loss
- Enhancing thickness

Types of Supplements

Biotin, fish oil pills, folic acid, multivitamins, and hair, skin, and nails vitamins are all types of supplements that can aid your hair growth. The following chart provides a breakdown of many of the benefits each of these supplements provides:

During the early phases of our hair journey, biotin was our supplement of choice. After about two short months of consistently taking the daily pills, we noticed many changes in the overall health of our hair. First, the pills almost immediately enhanced its overall shine. Then, we noticed improvements in the elasticity and strength of our hair. By the third month, we noticed our hair was becoming thicker than it had been in previous years.

We have heard multiple success stories surrounding supplements. Similarly, we have received letters and comments about poor results. Many of these stories however, are rooted in improper use of a product or the user's lack of patience.

A Kurly Confession

I have watched Kelsey and Kendra, now known as the GlamTwinz, since the time before they were on anyone's computer screen. In high school, they began to take what I thought was outlandish measures to protect and grow their hair. However, just a few months after their newly implemented hair care routine, I noticed the difference in the appearance and health of their hair. So, when their hair began to grow like crazy, I jumped on the wagon. Unfortunately, I had some catching up to do.

I started phoning them for hair tips and instructions. Whatever they said to do, I did it to the thirteenth power. So, when they said, "deep condition," I used the whole bottle; when they said, "let your conditioner sit for 30 minutes," I let it sit for three hours; and when they said, "take one biotin per day, I took two or three." Regrettably, while their hair kept growing, my hair remained stagnant and I could not figure out why. What was I doing wrong?

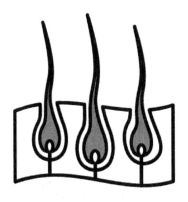

HAIR RECEIVES NUTRIENTS VIA BLOOD

BIOTIN

- ◊ Promotes Growth
- ◊ Boosts Growth Speed
- ◊ Prevents Dryness
- ◊ Prevents Breakage
- ◊ Enhances Elasticity
- ◊ Improves Thickness
- ◊ Refines Overall Health

FISH OIL PILLS

- ◊ Boosts Luminosity
- ◊ Increases Elasticity
- ◊ Improves Shine
- ◊ Improves Strength
- ◊ Prevents Breakage

FOLIC ACID

- Renews Hair Growth Cells
- Improves Growth
- Boosts Growth Speed
- Prevents Graying
- Promotes Luster
- Improves Shine

MULTIVITAMINS
(including Vitamin A, C, D, E, Iron, & Magnesium)

- Boosts Overall Growth
- Improves Thickness
- Minimizes Dryness

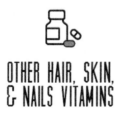

OTHER HAIR, SKIN, & NAILS VITAMINS

- Improves Shine
- Prevents Breakage
- Improves Thickness
- Enhances Luminosity

Then, one day while five or six of our family and friends were all sitting around talking, someone mentioned that she too had implemented the biotin in her hair routine and was experiencing great results. This was my golden opportunity—my opportunity to express my disdain about biotin and how it just did not work for me. Kendra asked which dosage I was using, and Kelsey immediately followed, asking how often I was taking it. "100 micrograms and I take two or three a day," I answered proudly. Their reaction was nothing like I had anticipated. Both Kelsey and Kendra began laughing uncontrollably.

"Two or three a day," they said in unison.
"They aren't candy," Kendra said.

"Yeah, and your body can only absorb so much at once. You are wasting them," Kelsey mocked.

"What do you mean wasting them? I had a lot of catching up to do. My hair was not growing!" I demanded.

"Yeah, but you can't rush it," Kelsey interrupted. "There are no shortcuts."

"Taking three will probably hurt more than it will help," Kendra added.

Then Kelsey explained, "Besides, after so much biotin is ingested, your body will just dispose of the rest."

After the conversation, I did a little online research and learned that the girls were speaking the truth. I cannot express how important it is follow the instructions provided by the supplement's label. In the end, it saves you time and money. Since then, I have been taking my biotin as recommended, using minimal product, and conditioning for the recommended period of time. My results have been incredible!

-Anonymous

The preceding "Kurly Confession" highlights a key aspect of supplement ingestion: at minimum, follow the directions as provided (nothing more nothing less). In addition, consider seeing a doctor (i.e. an endocrinologist or tricologist) before you select a supplement. You can request your doctor to perform a blood test to determine which key nutrients your body might be lacking. Comparing key nutrients provided by various supplements, along with blood test results will help you determine which supplement is best for you. It can also aide in helping you to know what dosage of your chosen supplement to take.

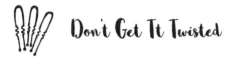 # Don't Get It Twisted

Although we are supplement endorsers, we do not guarantee that your results will be identical to ours or that because we selected Biotin you should select the same vitamin. What we are saying is that everyone's body is different. What one user may need, another may not. What works well for one user may not work as well for others. One supplement may give user one two inches of growth in the first two months, while the same supplement may give user two only one inch in the same time frame.

What we are saying is that the cells that penetrate the growth of your hair require nutrients—the proper balance of nutrients. Vitamins are a great way to supplement your body with any nutrients it may be lacking to propel your hair growth. However, understanding which supplement is right for you may take some trial and error. Nevertheless, with some consistency, your patience will be rewarded.

Consistency is Key

Taking supplements as directed daily is one of the easiest steps in your hair growth process. But in order for you to see realistic results, you must be consistent. The more you include supplements in your hair routine, the easier it will be to remain consistent. What's not to love about the benefits of a pill-sized capsule of nutrients that will improve and promote the look, health, and growth of your hair?! Supplements aren't mandatory for the hair growth process, but they remain one of the best methods in which people can see faster results.

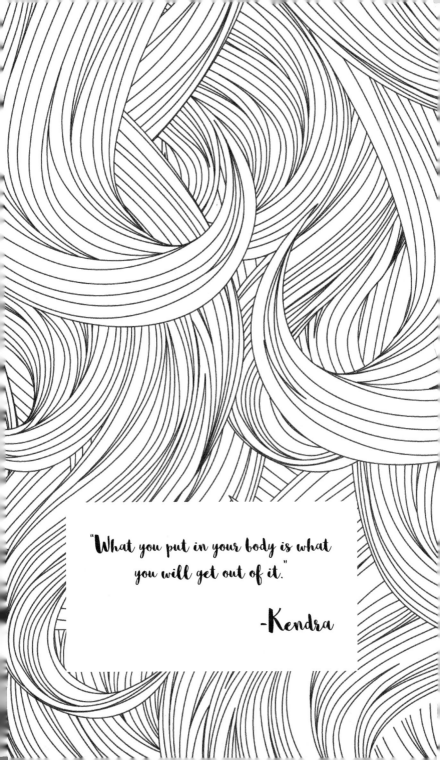

"What you put in your body is what you will get out of it."

-Kendra

CHAPTER 9:
LIVING HEALTHY

Cluuk, cluuk, pow. Lexi's car made a very distinct sound as it came to rest on the side of the freeway. Lexi, who was the proud owner of a slightly used luxury car, was devastated. It was the middle of the night, the area in which she sat was poorly lit, and her cell battery was low. As she dialed her fiancé's number, she hoped she had enough batter strength for an SOS call, but she was reluctant to tell him that her vehicle had stopped.

Over their three-year relationship, Daniel, a certified mechanic, repeatedly warned Lexi about the manner in which she cared for her car. He warned her that constant, abrupt stopping damaged the brake pads; improper and untimely oil changes impaired the engine; inadequate steering and stopping reduced tire life... the list was endless. Every time there was a problem with her car he could pin-point the action which had caused the problem. For instance, last year, when she needed new CV joint axles, he knew she had been making hard turns and jarring the steering column (whatever that meant). It was like the man had a car-enhanced crystal ball, and he was watching her every move, turn, and stop. So, she knew that when she explained that she was on the side of the road, he would know why.

When she purchased the car, he had cautioned her that a luxury car required a certain type of fuel. She was supposed to use premium gas. Unfortunately, every time she parked at the pump, she just could not bring herself to pay the almost $4-a-gallon premium price, when the gas labeled, '87', was closer to $3 per gallon. She figured a few regular, unleaded fill-ups here and there wouldn't hurt. Obviously, her hypothesis was far-fetched; after all, her car sat lifeless on the side of the road.

Just like Lexi's car required a certain type of gas for maximum performance, our bodies demand a certain level of nutrients for maximum hair growth and strength. When we fail to fuel our body with the proper source of nutrients, our hair growth halts—just like Lexi's car stalled. A healthy lifestyle is a convenient way to have and maintain healthy hair. What you put in your body is what you will get out of it.

Your hair (and nails) is made of keratin, a type of protein. When we replenish cells, it pushes dead cells toward your inner scalp. Those cells are shoved onto each follicle, and each follicle penetrates the scalp. As the new cells grow, the older cells die and are forced along the follicle, emerging as hair. Therefore, the more protein you eat, the stronger the cells; the stronger those cells, the sturdier the keratin; and the stronger the keratin, the healthier the strand. The pattern is cyclic, and the cycle begins with the foods and drinks we consume daily.

We bet you never thought your breakfast, lunch, and dinner could benefit your hair's health. Yes, you can "feed your hair." Putting the right things in your body will benefit you in more ways than one. Eating lots of fruits and veggies that contain biotin, vitamin C, potassium, and other nutrients are a great way to enhance the look, feel, and integrity of your hair.

Our Lifestyle

Lexi could not substitute premium gas with unleaded gas, and we cannot substitute pills, burgers, and sugars for naturally-occurring nutrients. If you watch our vlog channel, GlamTwinzTV, you know we are proponents of healthy living. We have found the benefits of healthy eating to be innumerous. A proper diet improves the appearance of skin, assists the management of weight, improves internal health, and produces incredible hair. Sure, supplements can fill a nutrient gap—but only to a certain point.

If you think you can eat potato chips and brownies all day and pop a pill to make up for the calcium, iron, zinc, protein and potassium your body craves, you are sadly mistaken. We cannot stress enough that there is no "magic pill" that can substitute these ingredients. That is precisely the reason why we suggest regularly incorporating nutrient-bearing foods in your diet. We have a few of our own favorites.

Foods We Love to Maintain Long, Healthy Hair:

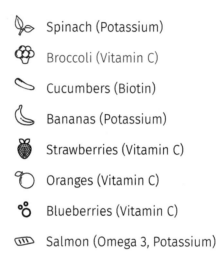

- Spinach (Potassium)
- Broccoli (Vitamin C)
- Cucumbers (Biotin)
- Bananas (Potassium)
- Strawberries (Vitamin C)
- Oranges (Vitamin C)
- Blueberries (Vitamin C)
- Salmon (Omega 3, Potassium)

Including foods like these in your everyday meals can help you achieve and maintain long, healthy hair. Each of these foods provides essential vitamins and nutrients your body needs to achieve maximum growth, strength, luminosity, and elasticity.

Better Foods...

While the idea of changing your diet sounds like a simple task, it may take some getting used to. Reforming your eating habits will mean more trips to the grocer, fewer trips to the fast food joint down the street, and more in-home food preparation. The task requires time, energy, and effort.

Many of the foods that increase hair growth and strength are naturally occurring—foods that grow from the ground and out of trees. The foods you want to incorporate in your diet are not processed in a plant and are not manufactured or packaged in a box. Fresh foods, like fruits and veggies, spoil over time if not consumed. Processed foods, on the other hand can sit on the shelf or in a box or a can, for weeks and months. Therefore, you will have to purchase many of these foods at your local grocer a couple of times per week.

More frequent trips to the grocer means fewer trips to convenient restaurants for a burger and fries. When we ate fast food regularly, we did so because it was a time saver. No food preparation or wait time. We drove up, ordered out, and ate fast. So, we know that healthier eating is more time consuming. To maximize our food prep time, we prepare an entire week of meals on a designated day.

On Sunday, we make the meals we plan to consume for Monday-Saturday. We leave ourselves one day without prepared meals so that we have three meals in the week during which we can eat out. This routine increases our discipline, encourages our routine, decreases any 'cheating,' and maintains our budget. Once you learn to make healthy eating fun, you'll see that it can enhance multiple areas of your life.

A Kurly Concoction

One of the ways we make healthy eating fun is by making smoothies! We love making them. We like to have daily smoothies that incorporate at least 2-3 of our favorite ingredients. For example, a strawberry, banana, and spinach smoothie is an easy and convenient way to include healthy ingredients in your daily eating habits. Smoothies can also be a good meal replacement and time saver for those who have hectic schedules.

Yes, this is the part of the book when we tell you the dreaded news—it's the same news your mom gave you ...the same instruction your doctor provided you... and the same advice that guy on TV told you... DRINK MORE WATER! Not drinking water can lead to major health problems. The lack of water can also lead to major dehydration. A dehydrated body means dehydrated hair, and dehydrated hair means dry brittle strands.

Not only does water make up a huge percentage of your body, but it is also the most beneficial thing to intake on a daily basis. Your body needs water; your hair needs water. There is simply no other way to say it. More H_2O, more H_2O, more H_2O. If we wanted to blow your mind, we would tell you to drink at least a gallon of water a day; Since we don't want to scare you, we won't tell you that (wink), but if you are drinking little to no water each day, you have to change that habit.

Of course, we have heard the day old excuse, "water tastes awful!" However, did you know that it is almost impossible for you to hate the taste of water. The water is not the problem (unless it's not clean water). The problem might be your taste buds. When we consume food and drinks with little nutrients, we reform our taste buds, and they adapt to those foods and beverages. Accordingly, when we eat and drink the healthy stuff, it can be unpleasant. It's almost like we flip flop our mouth's preference.

Don't worry, transforming your taste buds is easy. All you have to do is drink more water. Basically, some people don't like the taste of water because they are not drinking enough. So, if you're someone who does not like the taste of water—get used to it.

AREN'T YOU GLAM WE DIDN'T SAY BANANA?

INGREDIENTS

 1 cup of frozen strawberries

1 whole banana

1 handful of fresh spinach

1/2 cup of almond milk

DIRECTIONS

First, peel one banana, and break it into pieces.

Next, add the banana, spinach, strawberries, and almond milk in a blender cup.

Then, blend until smooth.

Finally, add additional ingredients for desired taste, if needed.

...MORE H₂O!

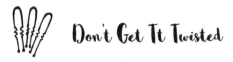 # Don't Get It Twisted

Do not misunderstand what we are communicating in this chapter. Do not expect to eat a banana today, and grow ten inches of hair tomorrow, and don't anticipate drinking a glass of water now and seeing shine and body ten minutes later. Healthy eating is not a one-meal-quick fix; it is a lifestyle change. The saying, "you are what you eat" is true. Eventually, your diet will tell on you. The people around you will be able to see what you consume in your weight, skin, hair, and nails.

Your diet is important. Calcium, biotin, Vitamin C, potassium, zinc, and protein are among the many nutrients your body will need to help you on your quest to long healthy hair, but changing your diet will not be an overnight feat. It will take consistency and dedication!

Consistency is Key

When we started drinking more water and eating better foods, we noticed our hair was a lot shinier and softer. Our skin was also noticeably clearer and more radiant. Water has numerous benefits, not only benefiting your body, but also your hair. Hence, the more you drink it, the more you'll like it, the better you will feel, and the better you'll look. Who doesn't want to physically feel better and have healthier hair? We believe in you. We know you can do this. . . so drink up!

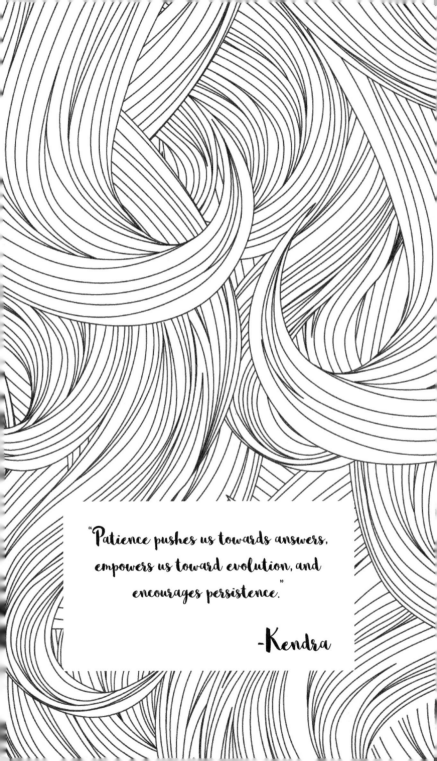

"Patience pushes us towards answers,
empowers us toward evolution, and
encourages persistence."

-Kendra

CHAPTER 10:
PATIENCE PLEASE

Whhhaaa!!!—it's the familiar, yet dreaded sound of a speechless, defenseless baby. The fact is, babies cry. They cry when they are hungry; they cry when they are wet; they cry when they are uncomfortable; they cry when they are cold; they cry when they are hot. Realistically, everything must be nearly perfect for most babies to remain calm and quiet. When things aren't calm and perfect, everyone around rushes to a crying baby, offering hugs, rocking, changing, and feeding to soothe the infant.

At birth, we perpetuate the need for instantaneous gratification. As a baby, crying infants are pacified; as a child, temper-tantrum-throwing toddlers are appeased (even if in the form of reprimand, the child is still appeased with attention); and as an adolescent, complaining teens are pacified. Our society enables impatience.

Even as adults, we wait on very little. If you want an instant meal, you can microwave it. If you want an instant answer, you just Google it. If you want a new purse, you can just charge it. We are losing the precious skill of waiting. Unfortunately, if you are one who has lost an appreciation for patience this journey may be a difficult pursuit, because patience is required for you to complete the quest for longer, healthier hair.

There is no way to cheat true natural hair growth. The only way to grow hair is to grow hair. Literally. There is no way to cheat the process. Hence, an impatient person will have a difficult time growing hair. The Kurly Confession in Chapter 8 shows that impatience may actually hinder the process.

When we are impatient, we are anxious, eager, and sometimes hasty. Anxious people make rash and irresponsible decisions. Consider a teenager who is used to getting all the latest fashions. When she shops, if she sees something she likes, she uses her parent-provided credit card to purchase it, but she has never worked a day in her life.

After college, when her parents inform her that she will now have to support herself, she will likely be unable to manage a meager budget. It may take some time for her to develop the skill of waiting and saving before making her purse purchases. In the meantime, she may spend rent-designated funds or max out a credit card making purchases to which she is accustomed.

Your hair is no different. Impatiently awaiting hair growth may cause you to take shortcuts or give up altogether—all of which can hinder hair growth or halt the progress. When progression stops, you may find yourself in the place in which you started or three steps behind where you could have been in the process.

On the other hand, if you are patient, you stand a better chance of making clear, conscious decisions. You won't mind making a budget to assist your new healthy lifestyle or to purchase the proper hair products. If you are patient you are empowered, because patience pushes us towards answers, patience empowers us toward evolution, and patience encourages persistence.

Being patient will probably be one of the hardest steps in this entire journey. Most people naturally want instant gratification. But having realistic expectations will get you through this process a lot easier. It took us around five years to meet our hair goals. We would be lying if we told you that it was easy. To aid your decision to be patient, we have put together a list of steps to help you on your way. Patience and these steps got us through this journey successfully:

1. Ask Why

Before you begin any journey, you must know where you are going and why you need to go. Let's first tackle why you want to go. Have you ever asked yourself, why do I want long hair? The answer doesn't have to be complicated. Maybe it's because you admire long hair, perhaps it's because it's been a lifelong goal, or maybe it's as simple as wanting to enhance your appearance. Take a moment to write your answer below:

goal. Will you be satisfied if your hair grows 10 inches long, 16 inches long, or 20 inches long? You may even answer the question without an exact number. For instance, we wanted to grow waist-length hair.

Jot your answer here _____.

2. Create an Image of Success

Now that you know where you are departing from, where you are going, and why you are going it should be easier to imagine yourself at your destination. Close your eyes for a moment (after reading this sentence of course), and imagine yourself achieving your personal hair goals.

Could you do it? Can you really imagine yourself with shoulder length, arm-pit length, or waist-length hair? If your answer is a definite, "yes," then you are well on your way. If you cannot see the image just yet, it is okay. Don't be discouraged. If you know that you cannot conceptualize yourself with longer hair, you must first understand that you will not maintain the patience to reach a goal that seems unachievable. So, you must put milestones in place to enable you to conceptualize the possibility.

(a) Achieving long, healthy hair is a long-term goal. If the goal seems too distant, it is often better to break it up a bit. For example, if you really want to achieve waist-length hair, first imagine yourself with healthy shoulder length hair. This image is likely easier to envision. Make armpit-length hair a second goal, waist-length hair a third goal, and so forth. We are not saying everyone should grow waist-length hair, but everyone can grow longer hair. Your goal will be personal, and the tips in this book can help you achieve it– whatever it might be.

(b) Also, it's okay to fake it until you make it. You can help your subconscious to visualize your hair goals. Find a picture of long healthy hair, cut it out, and paste it to a picture of yourself. Tape the picture to your bathroom mirror, and look at it every morning when you brush your teeth or wash your face. The goal is to see yourself at your destination point. It might seem silly, but these images will enable you to envision yourself at the end of the journey; it will encourage you.

3. Develop a plan

Having a plan is like having a map to get to your desired destination. You want to approach the tips in this book like a workout plan. Being impatient and inconsistent will prolong the entire process. Not being patient and being inconsistent will prolong the entire process. Just like working out, you can't expect change overnight.

Naturally, your map will be different from the next traveler because your hair requires a customized plan. Write down your plan. How often do you plan to deep condition? What days of the week do you intend to cleanse? How often will you moisturize? How often will you use heat? As you work the plan, you will begin to learn what works or doesn't work for your hair. Then, you can alter, modify, or update the plan as necessary. Include these tips in your normal, weekly, or bi-weekly schedule, like doing laundry or cleaning the house.

Making these tips routine, will make your routine feel like less of a hassle. Routines are something you do without thinking. Once you incorporate and follow the plan for a couple of months, it will seem like second nature. Your map will become your daily or weekly habit. On the next couple of pages, take some time to develop your personalized plan.

_____'S PLAN FOR LONG, HEALTHY HAIR

Insert Your Name

WHY I WANT LONGER, HEALTHIER HAIR

_____

_____

MY HAIR GOAL

_____

_____

TIME MY GOAL WILL TAKE TO ACHIEVE

_____

HOW OFTEN?	WEEKLY	BIWEEKLY	MONTHLY	AS NEEDED	OTHER

HEAT

WEARING
PROTECTIVE STYLES

WEAR LOOSE HAIR

CO-WASH

CONDITION

DEEP CONDITION

MOISTURIZE

TRIM

TAKE SUPPLEMENTS

Personal Notes

4. Find a Friend

Writing your plan will help you with step four—finding a friend. Achieving any goal is easier and more enjoyable with support. If you have support, when you feel tired someone else can take the wheel; and when you feel as if you just want to give up, they can remind you of why you started the journey.

We realized one thing . . . we had each other. Some might even say we were able to get results in half the time because we learned vicariously from each other. When one of us tried something and it didn't work, we were able to inform the other. And when one of us didn't feel like cleansing, the other was there to make sure we got up, cleansed our hair, and deep conditioned.

While everyone doesn't have a twin, everybody can make a friend. Partner an accountability friend. Give him or her a copy of this plan, and determine a day or time when he or she might call you for an update on your progress. You'll want to share your positive results and consistency with your accountability partner. This will encourage you to perform your plan as instructed.

5. Don't Give Up

Many people get discouraged in the middle of the journey. After all, patience is only required for obstacles or processes that take time. When we think of patience, we think of paint drying, rain falling, babies developing, plants growing, and pearls crystallizing. Although each of these processes take time, they always produce a beautiful result because anything worth having is worth the wait.

Growing longer, healthier hair is a journey. Journeys take time, and any time-consuming process requires patience. Patience encourages our ability to learn our hair and its needs. Patience also empowers self-faith to achieve our personal goals. Everyone's journey will be different. Our hair goals took five years to achieve. Your hair goal may require more or less time to achieve your personalized goal, but it can be done.

To aid your patience, develop a plan for your hair maintenance and care. Reading your plan often, following your routine regularly, and speaking with your accountability buddy frequently are all tools to help you remain consistent and encourage your patience. Don't give up, and remember, what's worth having won't come easily. Just don't overthink it and the results will come with time. We did it, and you can too!

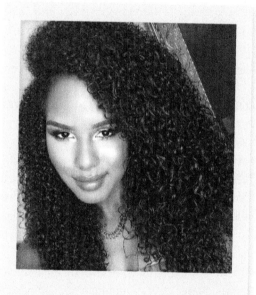

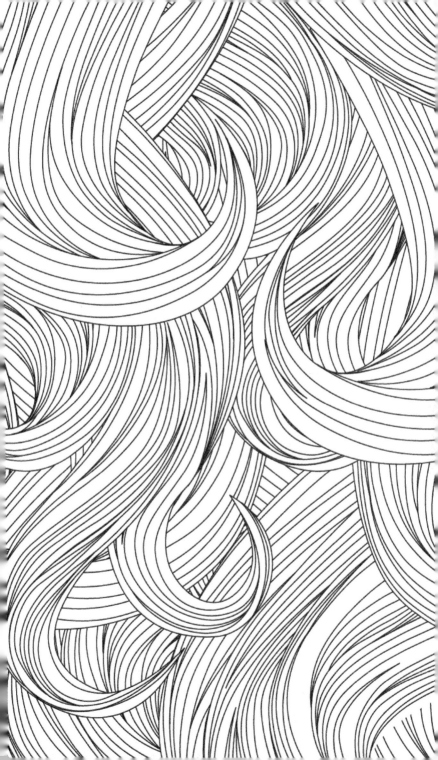

ACKNOWLEDGEMENTS

First and foremost, we would like to thank our Lord Jesus Christ for giving us "favor throughout our lives. We know that all good things come from Him and we are so blessed and incredibly grateful.

To our amazing mother, Josenca Murrell-Shaw, if it were not for you we would not be the independent, hardworking and driven women we are today. You are the true definition of a phenomenal women and we love you so much.

To our incredible grandparents, Joe & Ethel Murrell, Sr. thank you so much for believing in us and supporting everything that we set our minds to. We are so blessed to have such amazing grandparents.

To our genius of a cousin and also Friend, Kia Scott. Thank you so much for your creativity and contribution to this awesome book. We have always been inspired by your determination and intelligence. You are like the Big Sister we never had.

To Mahisha Dellinger (CURLS Founder & CEO), thank you for your willingness to writing the foreword without hesitation and contributing your business savvy advice. We are very appreciative and grateful for this and for our relationship with CURLS.

To Hugo Villabona and the editors, designers & publishers of Mango Media, thank you so much for giving us the opportunity to write our very first book and for taking a chance on us.

Last but not least, to our amazing subscribers and supporters, we thank you so much for your continued support and loyalty. Thank you for blessing us with a purpose to inspire. We hope that this book will help you achieve your hair goals.

AUTHOR BIO

Kelsey and Kendra Murrell, also known as the GlamTwinz, are spreading confidence to women and girls across the country. The Glamtwinz are certified Master Cosmetologists who specialize in hair and fashion. The glam duo are most known for their unprecedented YOUTUBE presence. With nearly 650,000 subscribers, over 400 videos, and 47,000,000 + video views across two YouTube channels (GlamTwinz334 and GlamtwinzTV) it's no surprise that the duo has partnered and worked with brand names like BET, Covergirl, Pantene, Dove, CLEAN&CLEAR©, Target, Ulta, Curls, Hairfinity, Carol's Daughter and so many others! Continue to watch out for these beauties as they continue to make their mark on the world!

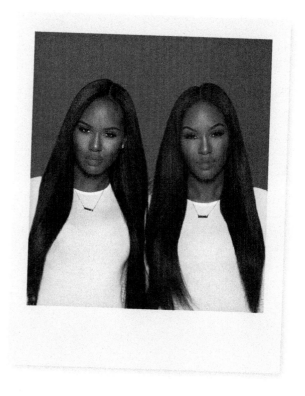

CPSIA information can be obtained
at www.ICGtesting.com
Printed in the USA
BVOW11s0011080616
451043BV00005BA/7/P